PreTest

Psychiatry

PreTest® Self-Assessment and Review

Notice

PRETEST

Psychiatry

PreTest® Self-Assessment and Review

Eighth Edition

Sherwyn M. Woods, M.D., Ph.D.
Professor of Psychiatry and Behavioral Science
Director, Student Psychiatric Health Service
Director, Psychoanalytic Education
University of Southern California School of Medicine
Los Angeles County/USC Medical Center
Los Angeles, California

McGraw-Hill Inc.
Health Professions Division
PreTest® Series

New York • St. Louis • San Francisco • Auckland • Bogotá
Caracas • Lisbon • London • Madrid • Mexico City • Milan • Montreal
New Delhi • San Juan • Singapore • Sydney • Tokyo • Toronto

McGraw-Hill

A Division of The ***McGraw-Hill*** *Companies*

Psychiatry: PreTest® Self-Assessment and Review, Eighth Edition
International Editions 1998

1 2 3 4 5 6 7 8 9 0 CWP PMP 20 9 8

The editors were John Dolan and Bruce MacGregor.
The production supervisor was Heather Munro.
Cover Designer was Jim Sullivan/RepoCat Graphics & Editoral Services.
This book was set in Times Roman by V & M Graphics.

Library of Congress Cataloging-in-Publication Data

Woods, Sherwyn M.
Psychiatry : PreTest self-assessment and review / Sherwyn M. Woods. – 8th ed.
p. cm.
Includes bibliographical references.
ISBN 0-07-052532-3
1. Psychiatry–Examinations, questions, etc. I. Title.
[DNLM: 1. Mental Disorders–examination questions. WM 18.2 W897p 1998]
RC457.5W66 1998
616.89'0076–dc21
DNLM/DLC
for Library of Congress 97-15680
CIP

When ordering this title, use ISBN 0-07-115870-7

Printed in Singapore

Contents

Preface

This eighth edition of *Psychiatry: PreTest Self-Assessment and Review®* has been extensively revised. The field of psychiatry has been covered in even greater breadth and depth with chapters oriented toward a developmental as well as a biopsychosocial focus on normal and disordered human behavior. The questions and explanations are consistent with standard terminology and definitions. K-type (multiple true-false) questions have been eliminated in keeping with the current trend in examination format. The questions and answers have been developed with an awareness that many readers will use this book to assess their knowledge while preparing for the United States Medical Licensing Examination (USMLE) Step 2 or Step 3. However, psychiatric residents will also find it useful in tracking the development of their knowledge base and in preparing for the PRITE examination.

I would like to express very special gratitude to my wife, Nancy Bricard Woods, for her patience, encouragement, and support.

Introduction

Psychiatry: PreTest® Self-Assessment and Review, 8/e, has been designed to provide medical students, psychiatric residents, psychiatrists, mental health professionals, and international medical graduates with a comprehensive and convenient instrument for self-assessment and review. The 500 questions provided have been designed to parallel the topics, format, and degree of difficulty of the questions contained in the United States Medical Licensing Examination (USMLE).

Each question in the book is accompanied by an answer, a paragraph explanation, and a specific page reference to a standard textbook or other major resource. These books have been carefully selected for their educational excellence and ready availability in most libraries. A bibliography that lists all the sources used in the book follows the last chapter. Diagnostic nomenclature is that of the fourth edition of *Diagnostic and Statistical Manual of Mental Disorders (DSM-IV).*

One effective way to use this book is to allow yourself one minute to answer each question in a given chapter and to mark your answer beside the question. By following this suggestion, you will be training yourself for the time limits commonly imposed by examinations.

Since there are few absolutes in clinical practice, remember to simply choose the best possible answer. There are no "trick" questions intended. Rather, each question has been designed to address a significant topic. Some important topics are deliberately duplicated in other sections of the book when this is deemed helpful. All questions apply to the treatment of adults unless otherwise indicated.

When you have finished answering the questions in a chapter, you should then spend as much time as you need to verify your answers and to absorb the explanations. Although you should pay special attention to the explanations for the questions you answered incorrectly, you should read every explanation. Each explanation is designed to reinforce and supplement the information tested by the question. When you identify a gap in your fund of knowledge, or if you simply need more information about a topic, you should consult and study the references indicated.

PRETEST

Psychiatry

PreTest®
Self-Assessment
and Review

Evaluation, Assessment, and Diagnosis

DIRECTIONS: Each item below contains a question or incomplete statement followed by suggested responses. Select the **one best** response to each question.

1. Psychological assessment can provide useful data in all the following areas EXCEPT

(A) symptom severity and change
(B) choice of medication
(C) cognitive functioning
(D) personality dynamics
(E) psychiatric research

2. A 40-year-old woman complains of fatigue, difficulty sleeping, and vague aches and pains and is preoccupied with her physical health. The clinical picture is consistent with all the following diagnoses EXCEPT

(A) occult carcinoma
(B) panic disorder
(C) endocrinopathy
(D) influenza
(E) depression

3. The most frequent indication for psychological testing in clinical psychiatry is to

(A) determine the correct dosage of medication
(B) determine the most effective psychotherapeutic style
(C) assist when there is uncertainty about the diagnosis
(D) assist in determining the length of treatment
(E) assist in generating clinical impressions

4. Evaluation of thyroid function may be particularly helpful in the diagnosis and treatment of which of the following conditions?

(A) Phobic disorder
(B) Schizotypal personality disorder
(C) Major depression
(D) Schizophrenia
(E) None of the above

5. The importance of an objective history is demonstrated in establishing the diagnosis of sleep apnea. The patient's bed partner, though not necessarily the patient, is likely to report all the following EXCEPT

(A) agitated behavior
(B) loud snoring
(C) sleep walking
(D) gasping
(E) bed wetting

6. Brain-imaging techniques, such as computed tomography (CT), would be most useful in evaluating

(A) bipolar disorder
(B) schizophrenia
(C) panic disorder
(D) Alzheimer dementia
(E) sleep apnea

7. Which of the following disorders has the most frequently positive family history?

(A) Post-traumatic stress disorder
(B) Social phobia
(C) Bipolar disorder
(D) Generalized anxiety disorder
(E) Somatoform disorder

8. Which of the following descriptions is true regarding persons who are at particular risk to commit suicide?

(A) They rarely communicate their intent
(B) They seldom have close family members who died by suicide
(C) They are almost always psychotic
(D) They rarely have a history of previous suicide attempts
(E) None of the above

9. A delusion can best be defined as

(A) false belief that meets specific psychological needs
(B) perceptual misrepresentation of a sensory image
(C) perceptual representation of a sound or object not actually present
(D) viewpoint able to be changed when convincing evidence to the contrary is presented
(E) dissociative reaction

10. In the United States the statistical suicide rate is higher in persons who are

(A) male rather than female
(B) single rather than divorced
(C) black rather than white
(D) married rather than widowed
(E) young rather than old

11. A 7-year-old girl hospitalized for a tonsillectomy awakens and cries out in fright that a "big bear" is in her room. She is relieved when a nurse, responding to her cry, enters the room and turns on the light, revealing the bear to be an armchair covered with a coat. This experience would be an example of

(A) a delusion
(B) a hallucination
(C) an illusion
(D) deja vu
(E) dissociative reaction

12. The parents of a 3-year-old child indicate that he seems to be clumsy, engages in hand-wringing, is poorly coordinated, has impaired language development, and a head that seems not to be growing in proportion to the rest of the body. The most likely diagnosis is

(A) Asperger's disorder
(B) porphyria
(C) attention-deficit/hyperactivity disorder
(D) Rett's disorder
(E) conduct disorder

13. In psychiatry, the electroencephalogram (EEG) has particular usefulness in the diagnosis of

(A) episodic rage reactions
(B) panic disorder
(C) schizophrenia
(D) social phobia
(E) frotteurism

14. Calculation of an IQ score requires knowledge of an examinee's

(A) mental age and educational level
(B) chronologic age and educational level
(C) mental age and chronologic age
(D) mental age, chronologic age, and educational level
(E) mental age and psychiatric history

15. An 18-year-old woman, previously in good health, seeks help at an emergency room for lightheadedness, headaches, and nausea. She appears anxious and is tremulous, sweating, and breathing heavily. While waiting to see a physician, she begins to complain of tingling around her mouth and in her fingertips. The physician should first

(A) ask her to breathe into a paper bag
(B) order immediate intravenous infusion of 50 ml of 50% glucose solution
(C) arrange for a brain scan
(D) conduct an amobarbital interview
(E) draw a blood sample to evaluate blood alcohol concentration

Items 16–17

As a part of the mental status examination, an interviewee is asked for the meaning of the proverb "People in glass houses should not throw stones." The person replies, "They will break the windows."

16. This response is an example of

(A) idiosyncratic thinking
(B) concrete thinking
(C) bizarre ideation
(D) loose associations
(E) none of the above

17. Patients who interpret proverbs in this way most often have a diagnosis of

(A) dysthymia
(B) paranoid personality disorder
(C) panic disorder
(D) passive aggressive personality disorder
(E) schizophrenia

18. All the following are projective tests EXCEPT

(A) Rorschach
(B) Hamilton
(C) thematic apperception test
(D) draw a human figure
(E) sentence completion

19. The Minnesota multiphasic personality inventory (MMPI) is

(A) a subjective test
(B) a projective test
(C) an intelligence test
(D) a personality test
(E) a special aptitude test

20. A 69-year-old man is suspected of having an acute onset of multiple small cerebral infarcts. The finding on mental status examination that would be most supportive of this diagnosis is

(A) a change in cognitive functioning
(B) depressed mood
(C) inappropriate affect
(D) delusional thinking
(E) anxiety

21. A psychiatrist finds himself annoyed with a quarrelsome patient for no apparent reason, and later notes that the patient reminds him of his quarrelsome and disliked sibling. This is an example of

(A) reaction formation
(B) projection
(C) countertransference
(D) identification with the aggressor
(E) illusion

Items 22–23

The format for the reporting of diagnoses detailed by the *Diagnostic and Statistical Manual of the American Psychiatric Association (DSM-IV)* is multiaxial. Each case is assessed along several axes, each of which is descriptive of a different class of information.

22. The presence of a personality disorder would be reported on

(A) axis I
(B) axis II
(C) axis III
(D) axis IV
(E) axis V

23. A physical illness that was relevant to either diagnosis or management would be reported on

(A) axis I
(B) axis II
(C) axis III
(D) axis IV
(E) axis V

24. The mental status examination includes all the following EXCEPT

(A) thought process
(B) mood and affect
(C) state of consciousness
(D) family history
(E) memory

25. The Halstead-Reitan test is used in the diagnostic assessment of

(A) personality disorders
(B) organic disorders
(C) mood disorders
(D) anxiety disorders
(E) sleep disorders

26. A person is sitting alone and behaving as if listening intently, then suddenly begins to nod and mutter aloud. This person most likely is experiencing

(A) a delusion
(B) an illusion
(C) a hallucination
(D) an idea of reference
(E) a flight of ideas

27. The condition of "waxy flexibility" is encountered during the physical examination of patients with

(A) alcoholic hallucinosis
(B) mania
(C) cocaine intoxication
(D) delirium tremens
(E) schizophrenia

28. The capacity to formulate concepts and generalize them is called

(A) concrete thinking
(B) abstract thinking
(C) delusional thinking
(D) intellectualization
(E) rationalization

DIRECTIONS: Each group of questions below consists of lettered options followed by numbered items. For each numbered item, select the appropriate lettered option(s). Each lettered option may be used once, more than once, or not at all. **Choose exactly the number of options indicated following each item.**

Items 29–33

Match each disorder with a symptom.

(A) Memory impairment
(B) Bizarre delusions
(C) Recurrent self-damaging acts
(D) Perfectionism
(E) Pathological jealousy

29. Paranoid personality disorder **(SELECT 1 SYMPTOM)**

30. Borderline personality disorder **(SELECT 1 SYMPTOM)**

31. Dementia **(SELECT 1 SYMPTOM)**

32. Schizophrenia **(SELECT 1 SYMPTOM)**

33. Obsessive-compulsive personality disorder **(SELECT 1 SYMPTOM)**

Items 34–37

Match each definition with the correct term.

(A) Prevalence
(B) Incidence
(C) Validity
(D) Primary prevention
(E) Secondary prevention

34. Early case finding and treatment to minimize duration of illness and to prevent permanent disability **(SELECT 1 TERM)**

35. The proportion of a population affected by a disorder at a given time **(SELECT 1 TERM)**

36. The proportion of a population that becomes affected by a disorder for the first time in a given period of time **(SELECT 1 TERM)**

37. Attempting to discover and eliminate the causes of mental illness **(SELECT 1 TERM)**

Items 38–41

Match each definition with the correct term.

(A) Magical thinking
(B) Blocking
(C) Looseness of associations
(D) Derealization
(E) Depersonalization

38. Discontinuous and illogical stream of thoughts **(SELECT 1 TERM)**

39. A belief that thought alone can result in the accomplishment of certain wishes or activities **(SELECT 1 TERM)**

40. Sudden cessation of thinking in the middle of a discussion or sentence **(SELECT 1 TERM)**

41. The feeling that one is standing apart from oneself and observing one's own actions **(SELECT 1 TERM)**

Items 42–45

Match each patient with the correct diagnosis.

(A) Mood disturbance
(B) Affect disturbance
(C) Disorientation
(D) Circumstantiality
(E) Tangentiality
(F) Perseveration
(G) Blocking

42. A 29-year-old patient describes witnessing a terrible plane crash that involved many victims and smiles and chuckles while telling the story **(SELECT 1 DIAGNOSIS)**

43. An adolescent patient responds to the examiner's question with the same response he has given to a variety of previous questions **(SELECT 1 DIAGNOSIS)**

44. A 75-year-old man is asked a question and gives a long answer that incorporates a great deal of tedious and unnecessary details **(SELECT 1 DIAGNOSIS)**

45. A 40-year-old woman shows little facial expression and states that she has been unremittently sad since the death of her dog **(SELECT 1 DIAGNOSIS)**

Evaluation, Assessment, and Diagnosis

Answers

1. The answer is B. *(Hales, 2/e, pp 247–272.)* There are many instruments available for psychological testing, and these produce useful data in a variety of areas, including symptom severity, cognitive functioning, and personality dynamics. The data are used in both clinical practice and research. The fact that these tests are standardized makes them particularly useful in conducting research. Psychological assessment is generally not used to attempt to resolve questions of choice of medication.

2. The answer is B. *(DSM-IV [see under American Psychiatric Association in Bibliography], pp 167–172, 201–202.)* Patient complaints of vague aches and pains and preoccupation with somatic complaints are particularly common to the diagnosis of depression. Often, depressed patients will present with such physical complaints rather than with psychological ones. It is important to remember that depression can also be associated with medical conditions such as occult malignancies or be a manifestation of an endocrinopathy, particularly Cushing's syndrome, hypothyroidism, and hyperparathyroidism. Viral illnesses can also be associated with a depressive syndrome. For these reasons, patients with depression should receive a thorough medical evaluation.

3. The answer is C. *(Hales, 2/e, pp 250–252.)* The most frequent reason for the use of psychological testing in a clinical psychiatric setting is assisting when there is uncertainty about diagnosis. Unlike semi-structured interviews that generate broad clinical impressions, psychological testing yields specific, comparable information about diagnosis and severity of symptoms. It is not useful in determining medications or dosages or length of treatment. No diagnosis should be made strictly on the results of testing, but these results are useful when confronting difficult diagnostic problems.

4. The answer is C. *(Yudofsky, 2/e, pp 524–526.)* Many of the signs and symptoms of hypothyroidism are similar to those seen in major depression, and thus thyroid testing is an important part of the differential diagnostic process. Some degree of hypothyroidism has been found in a significant percentage of both inpatients and outpatients being treated for depression. Thyroid testing should definitely be considered when depressed patients complain of a lack of energy, have symptoms or a family history of thyroid disorder, or fail to respond to antidepressant medication.

5. The answer is C. *(Hales, 2/e, pp 207, 841–842.)* An objective history from the spouse is of great importance in establishing the diagnosis of obstructive sleep apnea. While the patient may be unaware of it, loud snoring is frequently reported by the bed partner. These patients often thrash about and gasp at the end of a period of apnea. Bed wetting may occur on occasion. Sleep walking is not a feature of the diagnosis.

6. The answer is D. *(Kaplan, 6/e, pp 613–614.)* Brain-imaging techniques include x-ray, computed tomography (CT), emission tomography, nuclear magnetic resonance imaging (MRI), and positron emission tomography (PET). These techniques are widely employed in research studies of virtually all psychiatric conditions, but in most instances the findings do not have major diagnostic value. In the dementias, however, abnormalities on CT scan are present in a large number of patients, including those with dementias of the Alzheimer type. The findings are not specific enough to differentiate Alzheimer dementia from other senile dementias, or even at times from normal controls. The findings might be helpful in distinguishing dementia from the "pseudodementia" that may accompany severe depression.

7. The answer is C. *(Hales, 2/e, pp 56–59, 208–209.)* Studies have consistently shown that genetic factors are important in the etiology of many psychiatric conditions, including the mood disorders, schizophrenia, and most of the anxiety disorders. Family and twin studies have provided the best evidence of a genetic factor, though these studies are often difficult to interpret because of the problem of controlling for the psychosocial factors that may be perpetuated in families. A positive family history is particularly common in bipolar disorder and schizophrenia. The existence of a genetic factor in these illnesses is further supported by many studies of twins and adopted siblings.

8. The answer is E. *(Kaplan, 6/e, pp 1739–1740.)* The psychiatric history is of considerable usefulness in evaluating risk for suicide. Patients at particular risk are more likely to have a history of psychiatric disorder (especially depression) and family members who have committed suicide. A past suicide attempt is perhaps the best predictor of increased risk. While psychosis is a definite risk factor, the majority of successful suicides occur in persons who are not psychotic. Most commonly, patients who commit suicide have directly or subtly communicated their intent prior to the act.

9. The answer is A. *(Hales, 2/e, p 204.)* A delusion is a false belief that is not supported by fact and cannot be challenged successfully by logic or reason. Delusions are not randomly selected but rather develop as a defense against or support for specific thoughts or experiences; consequently, delusional thinking is said to be under the control of emotional, not rational, forces. What might be viewed as delusional to members of one social or cultural group may not be viewed as such by members of a widely divergent culture or social system.

10. The answer is A. *(Kaplan, 6/e, pp 1739–1740.)* In the United States it has been found that suicide rates increase with increasing age, and at all ages males commit suicide more often than females in ratios that range from 2:1 to 7:1. Married persons have the lowest suicide rate, with singles twice as apt, and widowed persons five times more likely to kill themselves. Blacks have a lower suicide rate than whites, and Jews and Catholics a lower rate than Protestants.

11. The answer is C. *(Hales, 2/e, p 213.)* An illusion is a misinterpretation of an actual sensory stimulus. A person's emotional state and personality needs can play an important role in determining the presence and type of an illusion. For example, perhaps the girl described in the question thought she saw a bear in her room because the hospital is a frightening, hostile environment for her. Systemic disease states associated with confusion (certain types of poisoning, for instance) also can produce misperceptions of sensory images by interfering with proper functioning of the brain.

12. The answer is D. *(DSM IV, p 59.)* Patients with Rett's disorder characteristically have normal prenatal and postnatal development until between ages 5 to 30 months, when they begin to lose previously acquired purposeful hand skills and develop stereotyped hand movements such as hand-wringing. They also display poorly coordinated gait or trunk movements and have severely impaired language development. A particular characteristic of this disorder is normal head circumference at birth, with a deceleration of head growth between 5 months and 4 years of age.

13. The answer is A. *(Yudofsky, 2/e, p. 237.)* The electroencephalogram has been used to study many psychiatric disorders, and particularly those associated with epilepsy and cognitive disorders. Clinically it is particularly useful and important in episodic impulse disorders, such as rage reactions. It may reveal organic pathology not easily demonstrated by other means. Abnormal EEG findings are not usually associated with the neuroses or with schizophrenia.

14. The answer is C. *(Hales, 2/e, p 113.)* IQ scores are determined by taking the ratio of mental age to chronologic age and multiplying by 100. This system of calculating the IQ was developed by W. L. Stern. The IQ is an indicator of relative brightness and can be used to compare children of different ages when mental age continues to increase in proportion to chronologic age.

15. The answer is A. *(Kaplan, 6/e, pp 1501–1503.)* The woman described in the question likely is experiencing a hyperventilation syndrome. Hyperventilation, which commonly is associated with acute anxiety reactions, causes excessive loss of carbon dioxide and, as a result, leads to respiratory alkalosis. As blood pH rises, ionization of calcium decreases, and clinical signs of tetany, such as painful muscle spasms in the hands, can become manifest. Other symptoms of hyperventilation include lightheadedness, headache, nausea, and tingling around the mouth and in the fingers and toes. Breathing into a paper bag reverses the symptoms because the reinspired air has a higher concentration of carbon dioxide than does normal air.

16–17. The answers are 16-B, 17-E. *(Kaplan, 6/e, pp 526–530.)* Part of the task of the mental status examination is to examine the patient for the presence of a thought disorder. An inability to form abstract concepts, illustrated by literal-mindedness, is demonstrated by the concrete interpretation of proverbs. It is a form of thought disorder called concrete thinking. Generally several proverbs are asked of the patient in order to make the determination. Concrete thinking is seen particularly in patients with organic brain disorder and also in patients with schizophrenia. It is definitely not a part of the clinical picture in personality disorders or in the neuroses.

18. The answer is B. *(Kaplan, 6/e, pp 551–584.)* Projective tests are standardized assessments that use unstructured situations to allow patients to "project" their personality dynamics and style in a non-threatening way. While the Rorschach is the best known, the thematic apperception test, draw a figure, and sentence completion tests are also widely used. The Hamilton is a rating scale used to assess symptoms and target behaviors in the evaluation of depression. It is not projective in nature.

19. The answer is D. *(Hales, 2/e, pp 252–253.)* The Minnesota multiphasic personality inventory (MMPI) is a questionnaire designed to measure various dimensions of personality. Examination of the responses rates the test subject according to nine clinical scales. Because it has been administered to large numbers of normal and emotionally disturbed subjects, considerable normative data are available. It can be administered to a large group of persons at one time and scored by computer.

20. The answer is A. *(Yudofsky, 2/e, pp 612–614.)* The possibility of an acute organic brain disorder mandates a careful examination of cognitive function. Acute conditions would be associated with a determination that the patient's cognitive ability had changed. For example, poor calculation skills in a person who had been a functioning accountant would be far more significant than the same findings in someone with a long history of poor school performance. It is the assessment of changes in cognitive function, rather than the specific cognitive disturbance, that is most crucial to a diagnosis of acute organic brain disorder. This is what helps the clinician to differentiate memory or other cognitive deficits of recent onset from those that are long standing.

21. The answer is C. *(Hales, 2/e, p 1040. Nersessian, p 438.)* Countertransference is the name given to the phenomenon when an interviewer develops feelings about an interviewee based on irrational and often unconscious factors. For example, countertransference may be initiated by the fact that the patient resembles someone in the interviewer's past. Sometimes these feelings are positive, and sometimes they are negative. When the physician or psychotherapist becomes aware of having feelings that are quantitatively or qualitatively inappropriate, it is wise to look for the presence of countertransference. Some analysts use the term more restrictively to refer to an analyst's inappropriate reactions to a patient's transference.

22–23. The answers are 22-B, 23-C. *(DSM-IV, pp 25–31.)* Axis I and axis II constitute the entire classification of mental disorders as defined by DSM-IV. Axis I consists of the clinical syndromes. Axis II lists both developmental disorders and personality disorders and can also be used to indicate specific personality traits or the habitual use of particular defense mechanisms. Multiple diagnoses can be recorded on both axis I and axis II. Axis III is used to record any current medical condition, physical disorder, or physical condition relevant to understanding or managing the case. So-called soft neurologic signs could be included here. Multiple diagnoses are permitted on this axis. Using these axes, a patient with depression might be recorded as follows: axis I—major depression, recurrent; axis II—narcissistic personality disorder; axis III—hypothyroidism.

24. The answer is D. *(Andreasen, 2/e, p 49.)* The mental status examination is a description of the mental functioning of a patient. It has a relatively standardized format. While the family history is an important element of the psychiatric history, it is not a part of the mental status examination.

25. The answer is B. *(Andreasen, 2/e, p 122.)* The Halstead-Reitan is a battery of five tests that provide a sophisticated evaluation of organic impairment of mental functioning. The reliability and validity of the test is well established. The time-consuming examination generally takes from 4 to 6 h.

26. The answer is C. *(Kaplan, 6/e, p 184. Andreasen, 2/e, pp 59–61.)* A hallucination is the perception of a stimulus when, in fact, no sensory stimulus is present. Hallucinations can be auditory, visual, tactile, gustatory, olfactory, or kinesthetic. Auditory hallucinations are most commonly associated with psychotic illness, whereas visual, tactile, gustatory, and olfactory hallucinations often are associated with neurologic disorders.

27. The answer is E. *(Kaplan, 6/e, p 539. Andreasen, 2/e, p 68.)* Waxy flexibility is a condition in which patients will maintain, for a long time, postures into which they are placed. When moving the patient's arms, a resistance is felt as if one were bending a wax rod. The condition is encountered in schizophrenia of the catatonic type. Patients with mania, alcoholic hallucinosis, delirium tremens or cocaine intoxication tend to be restless and/or hyperactive but do not demonstrate waxy flexibility.

28. The answer is B. *(Andreasen, 2/e, p 51.)* The capacity to generalize a concept is called abstract thinking The inability to abstract is called concreteness and is seen in organic disorders and sometimes in schizophrenia. The ability to do abstract thinking is commonly evaluated by testing similarities, differences, and the meaning of proverbs. Intellectualization and rationalization are mechanisms of defense, while delusional thinking refers to fixed beliefs with no basis in reality.

29–33. The answers are 29-E, 30-C, 31-A, 32-B, 33-D. *(DSM-IV, pp 274–279, 629–673.)* Paranoid personalities are often litigious and guarded and anticipate harm. They question the loyalty of others and therefore often are pathologically jealous. Transient psychotic symptoms may appear during severe stress.

The borderline personality disorder is characterized by emotional instability in a variety of areas, but particularly with regard to self-image and interpersonal relationships. These patients display unpredictable and impulsive behavior that may be potentially self-damaging. Stress-related paranoid ideation or severe dissociative symptoms may occur.

Dementia typically interferes with social or occupational functioning because it impairs memory as well as other cognitive functions. Changes in personality and behavior may also occur. The nature of the underlying cause will determine whether impairment is reversible or partially reversible.

Schizophrenia is a major psychotic illness that involves marked social, cognitive, and emotional dysfunction. Bizarre delusions are especially suggestive of schizophrenia, particularly in association with hallucinations. The illness may be associated with deterioration in level of functioning and includes both positive and negative signs and symptoms.

The obsessive-compulsive personality is often described as rigid, preoccupied with orderliness, and perfectionistic, as well as preoccupied with rules, details, and order. There may be difficulty in making decisions and scrupulousness about matters of ethics or morality.

34–37. The answers are 34-E, 35-A, 36-B, 37-D. *(Hales, 2/e, pp 86–91.)* All the terms listed in the question group are particularly common to psychiatric epidemiology. Prevalence studies in psychiatry are far more common than incidence studies. Prevalence equals the cases in the population divided by the total population (cases plus non-cases). It is generally measured at a given point in time (point prevalence) or over a given period of time (period prevalence). It counts both old and new cases, in contrast to incidence, which is a measure of the number of new cases that occur in a specified period.

Validity refers to the accuracy and verifiability of a study. It is usually demonstrated by agreement between two attempts to measure the same issue by different methods.

Primary prevention represents the attempt to discover and then eliminate the causes of illness, while secondary prevention relates to early case finding and treatment to shorten the illness and prevent permanent disability. Tertiary prevention is involved with rehabilitation.

38–41. The answers are 38-C, 39-A, 40-B, 41-E. *(Hales, 2/e, pp 204, 213–215.)* Looseness of associations refers to a string of thoughts that are disconnected in content and are illogical in their sequence. Circumstantiality is a disorder of association by which too little selective suppression of ideas allows too many associated concepts to come into consciousness. The connection between ideas, however, is usually logical and easy to follow.

Difficulty holding on to a train of thought—blocking—often manifests as an interruption in the middle of a thought. The sentence following such an interruption may have no relationship to what has just been said. Blocking, which is thought to be due to an intensification of anxiety, is not a conscious mechanism and thus not subject to conscious control.

Magical thinking is displayed by children, people affected by a variety of psychiatric conditions, and some primitive peoples. Essentially, it is a belief that specific thoughts, words, or gestures can directly lead to the fulfillment of wishes. Such thinking demonstrates an unrealistic understanding of the relationship between cause and effect.

Depersonalization is the sense of being outside one's own body, observing oneself as an actor engaged in a role. This symptom may be manifested by people suffering from temporary anxiety, neurotic (especially phobic) people, and severely mentally ill people, such as certain schizophrenics. Some people with an organic brain disorder, such as temporal lobe epilepsy, may develop both depersonalization and derealization, the feeling that one's surroundings are unfamiliar or unreal.

42–45. The answers are 42-B, 43-F, 44-D, 45-A. *(Hales, 2/e, pp 212–217.)* All the choices refer to elements that are attended to during the mental status examination. This examination is critical to the task of differential diagnosis.

Mood refers to the sustained feeling tone that exists over time for the patient. The patient may describe it, or the clinician may infer it from the patient's verbal and nonverbal behavior. Commonly encountered moods would include depressed, angry, euphoric, or anxious. Depression is often referred to as a mood disorder. Affect, on the other hand, is the feeling tone that accompanies the patient's verbalizations or immediate behaviors. In schizophrenia, affect is commonly found to be inappropriate or flat. Blunting of affect is commonly found in brain disorders.

Tangentiality is present when the patient's thought processes digress from the subject at hand to thoughts that are oblique or irrelevant. Circumstantiality is a disorder of associations wherein the patient lacks goal directedness and incorporates tedious and unnecessary details and has difficulty in reaching the point. In perseveration, the patient displays an inability to change the topic or repeats essentially the same response to a variety or questions or topics. In blocking, the patient will suddenly stop, usually in the middle of a sentence, and cannot complete his or her thoughts.

Disorientation represents the patient's inability to know who he is, where he is, the date or time, or the nature of the present circumstances. It is often found, for example, in the cognitive disorders and is important as a clue to the patient's ability to give informed consent.

Human Behavior: Theories of Personality and Development

DIRECTIONS: Each item below contains a question or incomplete statement followed by suggested responses. Select the **one best** response to each question.

46. Abraham Maslow interpreted personality in terms of

(A) motivation
(B) philosophy
(C) sexual development
(D) biological imperatives
(E) endocrine influences

47. True statements about personality traits include all the following EXCEPT

(A) they are tendencies to show consistent patterns of thoughts, feelings, and actions
(B) they are relatively enduring features that characterize the person
(C) they are synonymous with habits
(D) they are subject to assessment by psychological testing
(E) their distribution in a population approximates a bell-curve

48. The developmental theories of Margaret Mahler are associated with

(A) genetic field theory
(B) psychosexual maturation
(C) cognitive development
(D) ethologic development
(E) separation-individuation

49. "Stranger anxiety" typically appears in children at

(A) 3 weeks
(B) 2 months
(C) 6 months
(D) 1 year
(E) 2 years

50. In females, puberty generally

(A) occurs 2 years earlier than in boys
(B) is associated with menarche at age 15
(C) is first manifested by broadening of the hips
(D) does not appear before age 13
(E) is associated with a height spurt that occurs later than in boys

51. Modern psychoanalytic theory holds that narcissism is

(A) a pathologic state
(B) a normal part of human personality development
(C) the most frequent cause of hypersexuality
(D) first manifested during the oedipal period
(E) of little consequence except in children

52. The theories of Carl Jung include all the following concepts EXCEPT

(A) animus and anima
(B) libido as sexual energy
(C) collective unconscious
(D) archetypes
(E) the "shadow"

53. Which of the following theorists primarily focused on the maturation of the sense of self from the infantile fragility and fragmentation into the cohesive and stable structure of adulthood?

(A) Piaget
(B) Erikson
(C) Freud
(D) Klein
(E) Kohut

54. Of the following diagnoses, the median age of onset is earliest in

(A) bipolar disorder
(B) drug abuse/dependence
(C) major depression
(D) obsessive-compulsive disorder
(E) phobias

55. All the following statements about the psychoanalytic concept of the oedipal phase of development are true EXCEPT that

(A) it occurs between the phallic and the latency stages
(B) it is usually followed by identification with the parent of the same sex
(C) it occurs only in the development of children destined to become neurotic
(D) it is associated with the phenomenon of castration anxiety
(E) it occurs in both males and females

56. All the following statements about rapid eye movement (REM) sleep are true EXCEPT

(A) REM sleep is associated with hypotonia
(B) the amount of REM sleep declines between adolescence and old age
(C) REM sleep is the only state in which dreams occur
(D) a person is more apt to awaken after REM than non-REM (NREM) sleep
(E) penile erections commonly occur during REM sleep

57. While homosexuality remains a controversial subject within psychiatry, most contemporary psychiatrists consider it to be a

(A) personality disorder
(B) neurosis
(C) genetically based brain disorder
(D) form of pathologic sexuality
(E) variant of sexual preference

58. Sleepwalking is correctly characterized by all the following statements EXCEPT

(A) it occurs most frequently late in the sleep cycle
(B) it often disappears as the person reaches adolescence or adulthood
(C) it occurs during the same period of the sleep cycle as sleep terrors
(D) it is associated with difficulty in awakening the sleepwalker
(E) it is associated with full amnesia for the event

59. Identity diffusion, as described by Erik Erikson, occurs primarily during

(A) infancy
(B) childhood
(C) adolescence
(D) adulthood
(E) old age

60. In psychoanalytic theory the superego

(A) is totally unconscious
(B) is a defense mechanism
(C) functions to reduce guilt and shame
(D) contains the sexual and aggressive drives
(E) contains the ego-ideal

61. The early studies of Rene Spitz suggested that

(A) disturbed mothers are instrumental in causing behavioral problems in early infancy
(B) infants reared with little maternal contact are more susceptible to infections and behavioral problems
(C) infants reared in an institutional setting are likely to become autistic
(D) the number of toys available to infants is a crucial factor in their development
(E) environmental variables have little impact on the health of infants

62. Psychoanalytic theory describes the ego as a coherent system of functions, including all the following EXCEPT

(A) primary process thinking
(B) regulation of instinctual drives
(C) formation of relationships
(D) adaptation to reality
(E) speech

63. True statements about Freud's theory of infantile sexual development include all the following EXCEPT

(A) masturbation does not occur until the latency period
(B) sexuality begins early in infancy
(C) adult sexuality is affected by childhood sexuality
(D) neurosis is linked with disturbances in psychosexual development
(E) oral satisfaction is the earliest precursor of developmental sexuality

64. Battered and abused children are

(A) usually from poor families
(B) most frequently affected from ages 6 to 8
(C) commonly born to parents who were themselves abused
(D) most often abused by their fathers
(E) most frequently female

65. Piaget is best known for his theories and investigations of

(A) cognitive development
(B) affective component of development
(C) mood-related development
(D) motor development
(E) kinesthetic development

66. True statements about the latency stage of development include all the following EXCEPT

(A) it begins following the resolution of the Oedipus complex
(B) it is the phase in which identity crisis usually occurs
(C) it consolidates identification with the parent of the same sex
(D) it is often associated with some sexual awareness or activity
(E) it involves wider peer contact

67. Primary process thinking is

(A) typically conscious
(B) nonlogical and primitive
(C) absent during dreaming
(D) characteristic of the neuroses
(E) rational and well considered

68. Harry Stack Sullivan's theory of personality development was characterized by an emphasis on

(A) sexual development
(B) genetic determinism
(C) religious exposure
(D) interpersonal relations
(E) ego psychology

69. Genetic factors are considered to be of major significance in the etiology of all the following disorders EXCEPT

(A) bipolar disorder
(B) schizophrenia
(C) posttraumatic stress disorder
(D) Alzheimer's disease
(E) Tourette's syndrome

70. Erikson's developmental theories differed from Freud's in that Erikson placed greater emphasis on

(A) cultural factors in development
(B) the unconscious
(C) the superego
(D) sexuality
(E) genetics

71. True statements about Carl Rogers' theories include all the following EXCEPT

(A) he developed a therapy termed *client-centered*
(B) all humans tend toward self-actualization
(C) objective reality is secondary to personal subjective reality
(D) human nature is essentially amoral
(E) one's sense of worth is determined by consistency with the ideals of significant others

72. In psychoanalytic theory the anal phase of development, which occurs between approximately 1 and 3 years of age, is characterized by

(A) compliance
(B) depressive episodes
(C) striving for dependency
(D) use of the word "no"
(E) head banging

73. Sexual drive, when defined as the spontaneous manifestation of genital excitement, is believed by most clinicians to

(A) peak at an earlier age in women
(B) be generally strongest during young adulthood
(C) be virtually nonexistent after the age of 60
(D) be reduced by elevated prolactin
(E) be androgen-dependent only in the male

DIRECTIONS: Each group of questions below consists of lettered options followed by numbered items. For each numbered item, select the appropriate lettered option(s). Each lettered option may be used once, more than once, or not at all. **Choose exactly the number of options indicated following each item.**

Items 74–76

The concept of defenses is central to psychoanalytic theory. Match each of the definitions below to the defense mechanism being described.

(A) Acting out
(B) Rationalization
(C) Isolation
(D) Repression
(E) Sublimation

74. The unconscious exclusion of an idea or feeling from conscious awareness **(SELECT 1 MECHANISM)**

75. The intrapsychic separation of affect and mental content **(SELECT 1 MECHANISM)**

76. The direct behavioral expression of an unconscious impulse **(SELECT 1 MECHANISM)**

Items 77–80

Match the following definitions with the correct term.

(A) Core-gender identity
(B) Gender-role behavior
(C) Gender-role identity
(D) Sexual identity
(E) Sex print

77. The internal experience of sexual arousal patterns and self-labeling **(SELECT 1 TERM)**

78. The inner conviction that one is a male or one is a female **(SELECT 1 TERM)**

79. The person's self-evaluation of psychological maleness or femaleness **(SELECT 1 TERM)**

80. The objective patterns of sexuality **(SELECT 1 TERM)**

Items 81–84

For each age below, select the psychosocial crisis, as described by Erikson, with which it is most likely to be associated.

(A) Identity versus role confusion
(B) Generativity versus stagnation
(C) Integrity versus despair
(D) Initiative versus guilt
(E) Industry versus inferiority

81. 5 years of age **(SELECT 1 STAGE)**

82. 15 years of age **(SELECT 1 STAGE)**

83. 40 years of age **(SELECT 1 STAGE)**

84. 65 years of age **(SELECT 1 STAGE)**

Items 85–88

Match the following definitions with the appropriate concept.

(A) Neutralization
(B) Wish fulfillment
(C) Identification
(D) Secondary gain
(E) Overdetermination

85. The concept that a symptom may have a number of different origins and meanings **(SELECT 1 CONCEPT)**

86. The process by which libidinal and aggressive drives are mastered and provide conflict-free energy **(SELECT 1 CONCEPT)**

87. The benefit derived as a result of neurotic illness **(SELECT 1 CONCEPT)**

88. The unconscious process by which persons pattern themselves after others **(SELECT 1 CONCEPT)**

Items 89–92

For each psychic phenomenon or experience listed below, select the psychoanalytic theorist with whom it is most commonly associated.

(A) Sigmund Freud
(B) Harry Stack Sullivan
(C) John Bowlby
(D) Melanie Klein
(E) Carl Jung
(F) Heinz Kohut
(G) Erich Fromm

89. Signal anxiety as a result of conflict between the id, ego, and superego **(SELECT 1 NAME)**

90. Relationship problems determined by the occurrence of empathic failures and developmental arrests **(SELECT 1 NAME)**

91. Anxiety highly determined by developmental bonding and attachment behavior **(SELECT 1 NAME)**

92. Personality styles influenced by archetypal modes of experience **(SELECT 1 NAME)**

Human Behavior: Theories of Personality and Development

Answers

46. The answer is A. *(Kaplan, 6/e, p 511.)* Maslow interpreted personality in terms of motivations. He believed the person's whole life is organized around a hierarchy of needs. The lowest in the hierarchy were the physical needs (e.g., food, water, sex, sleep) and the highest were for such things as truth, beauty, and justice.

47. The answer is C. *(Kaplan, 6/e, pp 512–513.)* Personality traits are characterized by their consistency over time, and while they are durable, they are not immutable and may be changed or modified by life experience or psychotherapy. They differ from habits in that the latter are specific to a single situation or setting. There needs to be cross-situational consistency to infer a trait. Traits may be inferred from careful clinical observation or psychological assessment. In a given population, a trait (e.g., aggressiveness or extroversion) will generally show a normal distribution curve.

48. The answer is E. *(Hales, 2/e, pp 110–116.)* Margaret Mahler's theory of early infantile development stressed the child's movement from an original symbiotic and enmeshed stage with the mother toward individuation and autonomy. This includes the child's gradual recognition of the mother as a separate object, an important aspect of the child's ultimate move toward independence. Rene Spitz is associated with genetic field theory, and Freud originally proposed psychosexual maturation as the key element in the developmental process. John Bowlby attempted to meld psychoanalytic and ethological thinking.

49. The answer is C. *(Hales, 2/e, p 110.)* A wariness of strangers generally appears at about 6 months, and outright fear is not regularly observed until 8 to 12 months. Stranger anxiety is greater when a parent is absent, or the stranger appears abruptly or attempts to pick up the infant. Spitz considered stranger anxiety to be an important organizer of early infant development.

50. The answer is A. *(Hales, 2/e, pp 128–129.)* In females puberty generally occurs about 2 years earlier than in boys, and menarche is generally present by age 13, though sometimes as early as age 11. The female growth spurt peaks at about age 12, while in boys, it peaks at about age 14. The first sign of puberty is breast buds and then growth of axillary and pubic hair.

51. The answer is B. *(Nemiroff, pp 73–81.)* Narcissism, or self-love, is a major concept in modern psychoanalytic theory. It is viewed as a normal part of the development of all children, beginning in infancy. It can become a pathologic issue in the presence of developmental conflict or deficit. Although it ultimately may become linked to sexuality, in and of itself it does not imply genital sexuality. It may be a contributing factor in hypersexuality, but certainly is not the major cause in most cases. Narcissism is an important contributing factor in self-esteem and is of significance throughout the life cycle.

52. The answer is B. *(Hales, 2/e, pp 176–177.)* While Sigmund Freud believed that psychic energy (libido) was sexual in nature, Jung contended that it was much more general in form and not explicitly sexual or sensual. Jung believed that the unconscious included a collective unconscious that consisted of racial and cultural memories shared by all human beings. This collective unconscious included archetypes, which consisted of innate ideas, accrued over the ages, about such figures as mother, father, and hero. Jung believed that all persons had both masculine (animus) and feminine (anima) prototypes within them. The "shadow" was his term for the animal instincts that are our legacy in the evolution from lower animals.

53. The answer is E. *(Hales, 2/e, pp 163–164.)* Heinz Kohut developed a variant of psychoanalysis that has had a powerful influence on modern psychoanalytic treatment. He believed that psychic development was primarily organized around the developmental vicissitudes of the self, especially in the relationship to interactions with self-objects. The most important self-object of infancy is the mother. Freudian psychoanalysis postulated a sequence of psychosexual development that stressed unconscious conflict and the influence of sexual and aggressive drives. Erik Erikson elaborated the role of culture in shaping the meaning of these drives throughout the life cycle. Melanie Klein is associated with the object-relations school of psychoanalysis, especially a minute dissection of the early relationship of the child and mother. Piaget is particularly known for his work on the development of intellect.

54. The answer is E. *(Hales, 2/e, p 98.)* While most disorders have a wide range of possible age of onset, the median age has been determined for the major psychiatric disorders. Phobias have the earliest mean age of onset (13), and it is not unusual to find them in younger children. The mean age for drug abuse is 18, and the mean age for panic disorder, major depression (unipolar), and obsessive-compulsive disorder is 23 to 25.

55. The answer is C. *(Kaplan, 6/e, pp 443–444.)* According to psychoanalytic theory, the oedipal phase of development occurs in all male and female children. It occurs during the third to fifth years, that is, between the phallic and latency periods. It is related to the Oedipus complex—namely, sexual striving toward the parent of the opposite sex and jealous and murderous fantasies toward the parent of the same sex. Oedipal striving is normally abandoned in the male because of castration anxiety, and in the female because of mother's disapproval and father's failure to comply. In both cases, this leads to a period of more intense identification with the parent of the same sex.

56. The answer is C. *(Kaplan, 6/e, pp 80–87.)* Sleep is usually classified into REM and NREM sleep. Most adults have three to six dreams a night during an average of 1 to 2 h of REM sleep, but dreaming can also occur in NREM sleep. There is a greater likelihood of awakening after REM sleep. The proportion of REM sleep decreases with advancing age, and it is associated with hypotonia and penile tumescence.

57. The answer is E. *(Hales, 2/e, p 222.)* While homosexuality was formerly considered to be a sexual disorder, the current view of the American Psychiatric Association is that homosexuality should not be considered a mental disorder but rather a variant of sexual preference. This change was in part based on accumulated evidence that the rate and type of psychopathology is no different in homosexuals than in heterosexuals. The etiology of homosexuality remains obscure and controversial. Many psychiatrists believe there is a biologic tendency, which is then acted upon by psychological issues in the course of development.

58. The answer is A. *(Yudofsky, 2/e, p 436.)* Sleepwalking is classified with the parasomnias and is commonly found in children. Very often it disappears when the child reaches adolescence or adulthood. Both sleepwalking and sleep terrors occur during the first third of the night. Sleepwalkers are partially aroused and ambulatory, but hard to awaken. They are amnesic for the event.

59. The answer is C. *(Kaplan, 6/e, p 483.)* Erikson discussed at length the turbulence of adolescence, and the fact that it was a period of development wherein the individual was deeply involved in solidifying a sense of identity. Identity for Erikson included a continuity with one's past, a sense of sameness as well as a solid sense of self that includes goals, aims, and life style, as well as sexual identity. Identity diffusion, which occurs to some degree in all adolescents and most markedly in troubled adolescents, is characterized by confusion, insecurity, and aimlessness.

60. The answer is E. *(Kaplan, 6/e, pp 450–453.)* The superego in psychoanalytic theory is the "site" of the ego-ideal and the conscience. It sits in judgment of one's behavior and wishes and decides right versus wrong, good versus bad, virtuous versus shameful. While largely unconscious, it does have conscious elements. The unconscious aspect of the superego may produce guilt or shame about wishes and fantasies, not merely deeds. The id is the repository of the sexual and aggressive drives, and the ego is responsible for mounting the defense mechanisms.

61. The answer is B. *(Kaplan, 6/e, pp 1120, 2357, 2367.)* Rene Spitz's pioneering studies on the effects of institutionalization on infants compared three groups of children: those reared by their delinquent mothers in the nursery of a penal institution; those reared in a foundling home with no maternal contact; and those reared in two-parent home environments. The infants raised in the foundling home showed a markedly higher incidence of disease and developmental delay. The key factor that differentiated this group from the others was the lack of maternal contact and not the type of mothering, institutional setting, or play environment.

62. The answer is A. *(Kaplan, 6/e, pp 448–449. Nersessian, pp 61–62.)* The ego mediates between the person's id, which contains the primitive drives, and the outside world. It responds to internal and external stimuli by finding an action or behavior that will give maximum expression to the drives within the bounds of the superego and reality. Its functions include reality testing, regulation of defenses, and the establishment of relationships. The ego is associated with secondary process rather than primary process thinking.

63. The answer is A. *(Hales, 2/e, pp 149–150.)* Freud postulated that the foundations of adult sexuality begin in infancy and described three phases. The oral phase lasts for the first year to year and a half of life, during which an infant's needs, perceptions, and pleasures are centered on the mouth, lips, and tongue. Masturbation begins in infancy with oral and then anal pleasures, ultimately becoming genital during the phallic phase. Freud felt that psychosexual disturbances in infancy not only shaped adult sexual behavior but were instrumental in the development of neuroses.

64. The answer is C. *(Kaplan, 6/e, pp 2455–2469.)* Child abuse is found at all ages, but children less than 3 years of age are affected most frequently and most severely. It is found in both boys and girls, and mothers, more often than fathers, are the abusers. Abused children are often found to have parents who themselves were abused, and the families can be found in all socioeconomic strata.

65. The answer is A. *(Kaplan, 6/e, pp 291–300.)* Piaget was a pioneer in the investigation of intelligent behavior. His interest was primarily in the cognitive development of children, and the affective component of development was of lesser interest to him. He elaborated stages of cognitive development from the sensory motor intelligence of infants to the abstract operations and thinking that become important in early adolescence.

66. The answer is B. *(Kaplan, 6/e, p 444.)* Psychoanalytic theory postulated a latency stage of development that followed the resolution of the Oedipus complex and preceded puberty and adolescence. It was originally believed that sexual interests disappeared from consciousness during latency, though modern clinical observations show that not to be true. It is during latency that children consolidate their identity with play and through association with the parent of the same sex as well as through wider peer interaction. The phenomenon of identity crisis is associated usually with adolescence.

67. The answer is B. *(Kaplan, 6/e, pp 439, 644.)* Primary process thinking is primitive, nonlogical, and timeless. This thinking characterizes the unconscious and is present in dreams and active psychosis (not neurosis). It is driven by the pleasure principle and uses symbol, metaphor, displacement, and concretization.

68. The answer is D. *(Hales, 2/e, pp 179–180.)* Harry Stack Sullivan is best known for his theory of personality development, which emphasized the central importance of interpersonal relationships. He believed that the first 5 years of life were crucial but not immutable in shaping personality. Personality continues to develop and change throughout adolescence and into adulthood. He emphasized the influence of social position and condition on development.

69. The answer is C. *(Hales, 2/e, pp 51–68.)* Most investigators believe that a significant genetic component exists for bipolar disorder, schizophrenia, Alzheimer's disease, and Tourette's syndrome as well as a host of other psychiatric diagnoses. The genetic component most often creates a vulnerability acted upon by the developmental environment. The evidence for a genetic factor is less well developed in posttraumatic stress disorder, but may well turn out to be a factor of vulnerability.

70. The answer is A. *(Kaplan, 6/e, pp 478–485.)* Erikson and Freud were both psychoanalysts, and both acknowledged the role of the unconscious. However, Erikson's theories of personality development were more concerned with the influence of the social and cultural milieu. While Erikson acknowledged the important role of sexuality, it was less central to his theory.

71. The answer is D. *(Kaplan, 6/e, pp 511–512.)* Carl Rogers was a psychologist who developed "client-centered therapy" and a humanistic personality theory. He believed that persons tend toward actualization, and psychopathology represents a distortion of that process. Children develop their sense of self-worth based on whether they meet the ideals imposed by significant others, and thus their subjective reality is of much more influence than objective reality. He believed that human nature was essentially and inherently good. This was in contrast to Freud, who believed that needs were selfish and primitive and actualization would be catastrophic.

72. The answer is D. *(Kaplan, 6/e, p 443.)* According to Freudian psychoanalytic theory, the anal phase is characterized by noncompliance and a striving for early independence. This leads to the frequent use of the word "no," which defines the child as different and independent from the care-taker. This was the second phase of infantile sexuality in Freudian theory.

73. The answer is D. *(Kaplan, 6/e, pp 1296–1304. Nersessian, pp 68–72.)* Sexual desire can be clinically best understood as a composite of sexual drive, motivation, and aspiration. Sexual drive is an androgen-dependent system in both males and females. It has a frequency that varies over the life cycle and is generally strongest in adolescence. Many persons over the age of 60 continue to experience sexual drive, though reduced compared with earlier developmental phases. Most clinicians believe that sexual drive declines after the twenties in males and after the thirties for most females. Elevated prolactin levels from pituitary tumors or phenothiazine are associated with decreased sexual drive.

74–76. The answers are 74-D, 75-C, 76-A. *(Kaplan, 6/e, pp 450–452.)* Psychoanalytic theory postulates that every person, normal or neurotic, uses defenses. Some defenses, such as altruism (vicarious gratification by service to others) and sublimation (gratification of a potentially objectionable impulse by socially acceptable means), are considered to be mature and healthy. Repression, isolation, and rationalization are neurotic defenses. Repression, which plays a primary role in the pathogenesis of hysteria, involves the unconscious exclusion of a thought or feeling from conscious awareness. It is often associated with symbolic behavior representing expression of the repressed mental content. Isolation involves separating painful feelings from the thoughts provoking them. Both the thoughts and attendant affect may be excluded from awareness or the affect may be displaced onto a different thought altogether. Rationalization involves supporting unacceptable ideas or behavior by basically inaccurate but plausible explanations. Acting out is an immature defense in which an inner conflict can be partially and transiently relieved by unconscious expression in impulsive action.

77–80. The answers are 77-D, 78-A, 79-C, 80-E. *(Hales, 2/e, pp 653–654.)* Sexual identity refers to how a person subjectively experiences his or her sexual arousal patterns. It includes an awareness of what is experienced as erotic and desirable and is a part of one's overall sense of self. For example, a person who experiences both homosexual and heterosexual erotic arousal might consult a psychiatrist because of confusion about sexual identity.

Core-gender identity reflects a self-image of one's biologic sex. It therefore represents the person's self-designation as being female or male. Generally it corresponds to biologic sex, but it may be ambiguous in certain hermaphroditic conditions as well as in gender-identity disorders such as transsexualism.

Gender-role identity refers to a person's self-image and self-evaluation that results in a belief that "I am male" or "I am female." It develops well into adulthood and fluctuates sometimes as a reflection of the person's evaluation of feelings, behavior, and performance. It is closely connected to the degree to which one feels one has adequately met the prescribed cultural role.

The sex print refers to objective patterns of sexuality. It is more comprehensive than preference for a particular sexual object or a specific sexual activity, but it is the deep-rooted script that is most able to elicit erotic desire. It contributes to the person's sexual identity (subjective-self-labeling), but forms the objective patterns that determine the substance of the person's sexual fantasies and behavior.

81–84. The answers are 81-D, 82-A, 83-B, 84-C. *(Kaplan, 6/e, pp 481–484.)* Erikson described the personality development of humans in terms of eight major, sequential stages. While acknowledging Freud's psychosexual developmental theory, Erikson broadened the scope of his formulations by including social factors outside the parent-child triad, by shifting the emphasis from psychopathologic constructs to issues of normal growth and development, and by concluding that the process of development is a lifelong one. The resolution of each of the eight stages of development depends, Erikson said, on mastery of prior stages and influences the course of subsequent stages.

In the oral-sensory stage (the first year of life), trust versus mistrust is the important issue. In the second stage, corresponding to the Freudian anal period, successful resolution results in autonomy; problems in this stage can result in shame or self-doubt. The third stage lasts through the fifth year of life and parallels the Freudian period characterized by the emergence of the Oedipus complex. Erikson describes the task of this stage as the healthy growth initiative. During latency, years 6 to 11, industry versus inferiority is the important psychosocial crisis. Building on the autonomy and initiative of earlier stages, children approach the tasks of adult life. Whether industry flourishes or feelings of inferiority arise depends on children's interactions with teachers and peers, as well as with parents. Erikson's ideas about the development of identity during adolescence are particularly well known. He felt that, during this period, adolescents try to integrate and clarify their own identities in relation to their parents, peers, and members of the opposite sex; if they are unsuccessful, role confusion can result.

Although Freud believed that the reworking of the Oedipus complex in adolescence was the final stage of development, Erikson saw development continuing into adulthood. He saw intimacy versus isolation to be the primary crisis of young adults. During the years of middle age, generativity versus stagnation is the key issue. Erikson emphasized the importance not only of rearing children but also of engaging in activities to help others, particularly new generations. In the final stage, people reflect on their lives. Adequate resolution of the stages of intimacy and generativity provides contentment in this stage (integrity); poor resolution can foster despair and a debilitating fear of death.

85–88. The answers are 85-E, 86-A, 87-D, 88-C. *(Kaplan, 6/e, pp 449, 469–483.)* Each of the terms listed in the question describes a concept important to psychoanalytic theory. Neutralization is the term suggested by Heinz Hartmann to describe the process by which libidinal and aggressive drives are mastered, thus freeing energy for the ego. This concept is important in helping to explain non-defensive ego functioning. Overdetermination describes the concept that mental phenomena, such as neurotic symptoms and dreams, have multiple causes and thus have multiple meanings.

Identification is a defense that plays an important role in normal development. It involves unconscious patterning after another person that produces structural change in the ego.

Primary gain refers to the relief of tension and conflict produced by the development of neurotic symptoms. In addition to the internal reduction of distress, neurotic persons may attempt to derive compensation or gratification from the external world (secondary gain) as a result of their suffering. Examples of secondary gain include an increase in attention and sympathy, relief from burdensome obligations, and monetary compensation.

Wish fulfillment is the term used by Freud to describe the primary goal of dreams.

89–92. The answers are 89-A, 90-F, 91-C, 92-E. *(Kaplan, 6/e, pp 143–182.)* In the structural theory, Freud proposed three divisions of the mind: id, ego, and superego. This was an advance over the topographical theory, which elaborated the concepts of the conscious and unconscious. The id is the site of the pleasure-oriented drives; the ego is the central mediating agency charged with interfacing with the id, the superego (conscience and ideals), and reality. Conflict, generating signal anxiety, occurs when unacceptable id impulses threaten to become conscious or to result in behavior unacceptable to the superego and ego.

Heinz Kohut was originally a classical psychoanalyst who later developed a system of psychoanalysis that is most often referred to as self-psychology. Rather than focusing on instincts and conflict, Kohut stressed the development of the self, particularly as it relates to developmental deficits and failures in phase-appropriate empathy. The development of a cohesive sense of self and self-esteem is seen as the most critical developmental task.

John Bowlby is usually classified among the psychoanalytic developmentalists. His studies suggest a primary bonding drive with age-related phases particularly important during infancy. This is expressed in attachment behavior consisting of clinging, sucking, following, crying, and smiling. He made the parent-child relationship central and not subservient to drive discharge.

Carl Jung was originally a member of Freud's inner circle, but later split with him largely over questions of libido, psychic energy, and the nature of the unconscious. Jung believed the unconscious was more than the product of personal history but also included a collective unconscious with memories of our cultural past, racial memory, and even prehuman memory. The unconscious contains archetypes, which are innate ideas that have accumulated over generations and then interact with life experiences. Archetypes include innate ideas about such things as mother, father, hero, and the masculine and feminine prototypes within us.

Human Behavior: Biologic and Related Sciences

DIRECTIONS: Each item below contains a question or incomplete statement followed by suggested responses. Select the **one best** response to each question.

93. Benzodiazepines, barbiturates, many anticonvulsants, and probably ethyl alcohol exert their influence through which of the following types of receptors?

(A) Muscarinic
(B) Dopamine
(C) Glutamate
(D) Adrenergic
(E) Gamma-aminobutyric acid (GABA)

94. Seasonal circadian rhythm has been implicated in the etiology of

(A) depression
(B) sociopathy
(C) Capgras' syndrome
(D) panic disorder
(E) obsessive-compulsive disorder

95. The classic epidemiologic research known as the Midtown Manhattan Study indicated that the percentage of the population that can be deemed "mentally healthy" is

(A) 5
(B) 20
(C) 40
(D) 50
(E) 75

96. True statements about amphetamines include all the following EXCEPT

(A) they cause release of dopamine at the nerve ending
(B) they inhibit dopamine reuptake
(C) they produce subjective effects similar to those of cocaine
(D) they increase hunger
(E) they are extensively metabolized in the liver

97. In the brain, transmission along the neuron and across synapses is accomplished by which of the following mechanisms?

(A) Mechanical
(B) Neurohormonal and mechanical
(C) Chemical
(D) Chemical and electrical
(E) Electromagnetic

98. The state of cataplexy

(A) may be precipitated by an orgasm
(B) is associated with unconsciousness
(C) involves a sudden increase in general muscle tone
(D) often lasts for 1 to 2 h
(E) is usually treated with neuroleptics

99. Hypothalamic function is closely related to all the following EXCEPT

(A) sleep
(B) appetite
(C) memory
(D) sexual behavior
(E) fear

100. The locus coeruleus is associated with

(A) noradrenergic neurons
(B) serotonergic neurons
(C) dopaminergic neurons
(D) GABAergic neurons
(E) cerebellar granule cells

101. True statements about beta-endorphins include all the following EXCEPT

(A) they are involved in the perception of pain
(B) they are released from the pituitary in response to stress
(C) they are classified as neurotransmitters
(D) they are highly localized to the cerebral cortex
(E) chemically they are peptides

102. All the following evidence supports the dopamine hypothesis of schizophrenia EXCEPT

(A) the largest concentrations of dopamine are found in the cerebral cortex
(B) the basal ganglia may be metabolically hyperactive in unmedicated schizophrenia
(C) the phenothiazine drugs block dopamine receptors
(D) many of the antipsychotic drugs increase the level of dopamine metabolites
(E) parkinsonism is a side effect of many antipsychotic medications

103. Most studies suggest that the major inhibitory neurotransmitter in the brain is

(A) serotonin
(B) dopamine
(C) beta-endorphin
(D) gamma-aminobutyric acid
(E) somatostatin

104. The Klüver-Bucy syndrome is characterized by

(A) compulsive anal activity
(B) rage attacks
(C) hypersexuality
(D) hypophagia
(E) catalepsy

105. Monoamine oxidase (MAO) inhibitors used in the treatment of depression exert their influence primarily by

(A) increasing GABA production
(B) blocking inactivation of biogenic amines
(C) decreasing norepinephrine
(D) decreasing serotonin
(E) increasing endorphin production

106. Typical behavior in patients displaying the catastrophic reaction, as defined by Goldstein (1939) and Gainotti (1972), includes all the following EXCEPT

(A) restlessness and hypermotility
(B) ingratiating behavior toward the examiner
(C) sudden bursts of tears
(D) cursing
(E) refusal to continue the examination

107. The dietary amino-acid precursor of catecholamines is

(A) tryptophan
(B) glutamic acid
(C) aspartic acid
(D) tyrosine
(E) glycine

108. The orbitofrontal syndrome, associated with injury or tumor of the frontal lobes, is characterized by all the following EXCEPT

(A) apathy
(B) irritability
(C) jocular affect and euphoria
(D) impulsive behavior
(E) emotional lability

109. While psychosis plus delirium can be found in a wide variety of severe endocrinopathies, psychosis with a clear sensorium is most likely to be found in

(A) hypothyroidism
(B) hyperthyroidism
(C) hypoparathyroidism
(D) hyperparathyroidism
(E) hypercortisolism

110. The cell bodies of serotonin-releasing neurons are located in an area of the brain known as the

(A) raphe nuclei
(B) locus ceruleus
(C) cingulate cortex
(D) basal forebrain
(E) frontal cortex

111. For a substance to be classified as a neurotransmitter, all the following must be true EXCEPT

(A) the substance must be concentrated in the presynaptic nerve terminal
(B) the substance must be released by a depolarizing stimulus applied to the neuron
(C) the effects on the postsynaptic receptor are the same whether the substance is released from the presynaptic neuron or applied exogenously
(D) the neuron must be able to synthesize the substance
(E) there must be no mechanism for inactivation of the substance after its release from the presynaptic nerve terminal

112. Which of the following types of studies offers the most promise in elucidating the interaction between genetic and environmental factors in psychiatric illness?

(A) Family risk studies
(B) Twin studies
(C) Adoption studies
(D) Genetic marker studies
(E) Prospective longitudinal studies

113. Information is transmitted along a neuron in a series of electrochemical events known as

(A) translators
(B) resting potentials
(C) action potentials
(D) polarity maintainers
(E) none of the above

114. The group of neurotransmitters known as biogenic amines include all the following EXCEPT

(A) gamma-aminobutyric acid (GABA)
(B) serotonin
(C) dopamine
(D) acetylcholine
(E) epinephrine

115. During REM sleep all the following occur EXCEPT

(A) variable or increased heart rate
(B) variable or increased blood pressure
(C) penile erections
(D) absence of dreaming
(E) decreased skeletal muscle tone

116. Non-REM (NREM) sleep is commonly associated with

(A) increased blood pressure
(B) increased heart rate
(C) frequent penile erections
(D) frequent dreaming
(E) night terrors

117. The biochemical model of obsessive-compulsive disorder implicates the neurotransmitter

(A) serotonin
(B) norepinephrine
(C) dopamine
(D) acetylcholine
(E) histamine

DIRECTIONS: Each group of questions below consists of lettered options followed by numbered items. For each numbered item, select the appropriate lettered option(s). Each lettered option may be used once, more than once, or not at all. **Choose exactly the number of options indicated following each item.**

Items 118–121

For each chemical classification, select the CNS neurotransmitter that is an example of that classification.

(A) Glutamic acid
(B) Gamma-aminobutyric acid (GABA)
(C) Norepinephrine
(D) Somatostatin
(E) Lactic acid

118. Biogenic amine **(SELECT 1 NEUROTRANSMITTER)**

119. Excitatory amino acid **(SELECT 1 NEUROTRANSMITTER)**

120. Neuropeptide **(SELECT 1 NEUROTRANSMITTER)**

121. Inhibitory amino acid **(SELECT 1 NEUROTRANSMITTER)**

Items 122–126

For each function described below, select the hypothalamic nucleus most likely responsible.

(A) Anterior
(B) Ventromedial
(C) Lateral
(D) Posterior
(E) Supraoptic

122. Acts as a satiety center for appetite **(SELECT 1 NUCLEUS)**

123. Stimulates appetite **(SELECT 1 NUCLEUS)**

124. Functions with the reticular activating system to control arousal **(SELECT 1 NUCLEUS)**

125. Influences sexual behavior **(SELECT 1 NUCLEUS)**

126. Produces antidiuretic hormone **(SELECT 1 NUCLEUS)**

Items 127–128

Match each treatment method with the substance for which it is a generally recommended means of overdose elimination.

(A) alcohol
(B) cocaine
(C) hypnotic
(D) opioid
(E) carbon monoxide

127. Administration of ipecac
(SELECT 1 SUBSTANCE)

128. Hemodialysis
(SELECT 1 SUBSTANCE)

Items 129–132

Match each substance with the major medical complication seen in overdose.

(A) Hypertension and nystagmus
(B) Respiratory depression
(C) Seizures and acidosis
(D) Cardiac and anticholinergic side effects, and hypotension
(E) Liver toxicity peaking at 72 to 96 h

129. Cocaine
(SELECT 1 COMPLICATION)

130. Phencyclidine
(SELECT 1 COMPLICATION)

131. Tricyclic antidepressant
(SELECT 1 COMPLICATION)

132. Acetaminophen
(SELECT 1 COMPLICATION)

Human Behavior: Biologic and Related Sciences

Answers

93. The answer is E. *(Hales, 2/e, p 21.)* The GABA receptors are especially important in psychopharmacology. The benzodiazepines, barbiturates, many anticonvulsants, and possibly ethyl alcohol exert their primary effects through activation of the GABA receptors. GABA is an amino acid. GABAergic neurons are localized to a large number of different neuronal systems throughout the brain.

94. The answer is A. *(Kaplan, 6/e, pp 134–135.)* Seasonal circadian rhythm has been implicated in the etiology of seasonal depressive disorder. It is hypothesized that winter depression is triggered by seasonal changes in the photoperiod, which in turn induces changes in the duration of nocturnal melatonin secretion. Patients with this disorder are often treated with exposure to light.

95. The answer is B. *(Hales, 2/e, p 94.)* The Midtown Manhattan Study sampled 1660 persons by structured interviews, interpreted by two psychiatrists. There was much skepticism about the findings. The study found that 81.5 percent of the population had at least mild impairment and 23.4 percent had significant impairment from psychological symptoms. This meant that slightly less than 20 percent of the population were "mentally healthy."

96. The answer is D. *(Kaplan, 6/e, pp 794–795.)* Amphetamines are central nervous system stimulants. They cause increased dopamine at the synaptic junction. The subjective effects and the toxicity are quite similar to those of cocaine. Both produce decreased hunger and decreased need for sleep. Amphetamines are extensively metabolized in the liver.

97. The answer is D. *(Hales, 2/e, p 3.)* In the human brain, electrical impulses trigger chemical events at the synapse. The release of presynaptic neurotransmitters stimulates postsynaptic receptors, and thus neuronal transmission proceeds across the synapse. The synaptic communication is primarily chemical, and this allows for the continuation of electrical impulses along the neuron.

98. The answer is A. *(Kaplan, 6/e, pp 641–643, 1376.)* Cataplexy involves an acute onset of profound, generalized muscular weakness that leads to collapse. The patient has full consciousness, and the attack is often precipitated by an unusual state of emotional arousal, such as great laughter or an orgasm. It generally lasts seconds to minutes. Neuroleptics are not used in its treatment.

99. The answer is C. *(Kaplan, 6/e, pp 22–23.)* Lesioning and stimulation studies have shown that the hypothalamus exerts control over sleep, appetite, and sexual and emotional behavior. Hypothalamic hormones and other bloodborne factors can influence behavior; moreover, the release and action of these substances are affected by the neurotransmitters—norepinephrine, serotonin, and dopamine—that mediate behavior. Memory is a complex function that involves cortical and subcortical structures and is affected by hypothalamic activity only in a secondary way.

100. The answer is A. *(Hales, 2/e, pp 16–23, 503.)* The locus coeruleus is located bilaterally in the dorsal pons. It is the principal noradrenergic nucleus and is the primary source of noradrenergic innervation for most of the central nervous system. It is believed by some researchers to be involved in the etiology of panic attacks.

101. The answer is D. *(Hales, 2/e, pp 22–23.)* The endorphins are endogenous opioid peptides that are highly distributed throughout the brain. Their discovery led to the identification of a number of peptides that are believed to serve as neurotransmitters. Beta-endorphin is of importance in psychiatry because it is released by the pituitary in response to stress and has an important role in the perception of pain.

102. The answer is A. *(Yudofsky, 2/e, p 632.)* The largest concentrations of dopamine are found in the basal ganglia. Positron emission tomography (PET) has suggested that the basal ganglia area may be hyperactive in schizophrenia. The dopamine hypothesis is also supported by the fact that nearly all effective antipsychotic medications block dopamine receptors, which results in increased production of dopamine and increased dopamine metabolites. Parkinson's disease is a side effect of antipsychotic drugs such as the phenothiazines and is associated with dopamine deficiency in the brain.

103. The answer is D. *(Yudofsky, 2/e, pp 10–11, 690–691.)* Gamma-aminobutyric acid (GABA) is believed to be the major inhibitory neurotransmitter in the central nervous system. It has an important role in modulating the activity of other neurotransmitters. Many investigators believe that it has an important role in the etiology of anxiety disorders, though the exact mechanisms are still speculative.

104. The answer is C. *(Yudofsky, 2/e, pp 108, 608.)* The Klüver-Bucy syndrome is related to bilateral temporal pathology. It is associated with compulsive oral activity, hypersexuality, docility, and hyperphagia. These patients often have an inability to ignore stimuli and may carry on a running commentary about all they see. The syndrome can be demonstrated in monkeys after bilateral temporal lobectomy. It may occur in fragmentary form in the late stages of Alzheimer's disease.

105. The answer is B. *(Hales, 2/e, pp 925–926.)* Monoamine oxidase inactivates biogenic amines such as norepinephrine, serotonin, dopamine, and tyramine through oxidative deamination. The MAO inhibitors block this inactivation, thereby increasing the availability of these neurotransmitters for synaptic release. Norepinephrine and serotonin have been hypothesized to play an important role in the pathophysiology of depression.

106. The answer is B. *(Yudofsky, 2/e, pp 450–451.)* In 1939 Goldstein was the first to describe the catastrophic reaction, first noted with patients with brain disease. It consists of an emotional outburst that typically may involve anger, depression, tears, refusal, shouting, or sometimes aggressive behavior. This is in response to physical damage to the brain (reported more frequently among patients with left hemispheric lesions and aphasia) or as a psychological reaction to severe physical or cognitive impairment. These patients are typically angry or aggressive toward the examiner and the examination that is provoking the response.

107. The answer is D. *(Kaplan, 6/e, p 25.)* The amino acid tyrosine is the precursor in the synthesis of dopamine and norepinephrine. Tyrosine is converted to 3,4-dihydroxyphenylalanine (dopa), which is then decarboxylated to dopamine. Through the action of the enzyme dopamine-hydroxylase, dopamine is converted to norepinephrine. According to current biochemical theories, this pathway is of critical importance in the pathogenesis of depression.

108. The answer is A. *(Yudofsky, 2/e, pp 480–481.)* Patients with an orbitofrontal syndrome have been called "pseudopsychopathic" because of their disinhibited and impulsive behavior, emotional lability, and irritability. They often display a jocular affect and euphoria. By contrast patients with injury to the frontal convexities often present with apathy, indifference, and psychomotor retardation and have been referred to as "pseudodepressed." While such distinct syndromes occur, frontal lobe tumors generally present with a mixture of symptoms, since various portions of the frontal lobes may be affected by extension, pressure, or edema.

109. The answer is D. *(Yudofsky, 2/e, pp 522–530.)* Virtually all the endocrinopathies may be associated with delirium and psychosis. This may also occur in hyperparathyroidism when calcium levels rise, and the delirium is usually associated with hallucinations and delusions. However, acute paranoid states, with or without depression and in the presence of a clear sensorium, have been reported in patients with hyperparathyroidism. Such patients may become suicidal, violent, and even homicidal.

110. The answer is A. *(Hales, 2/e, pp 27–28.)* The cell bodies of serotonin-releasing neurons are located in the midbrain in a group of nuclei called the raphe nuclei. These neurons provide innervation to essentially all areas of the central nervous system.

111. The answer is E. *(Yudofsky, 2/e, pp 7–18.)* Neurotransmitters are chemical messengers that transfer information between neurons, i.e., from pre- to postsynaptic neurons. To be designated as a neurotransmitter, a substance must satisfy a number of criteria. These criteria include the necessity for a mechanism to inactivate the neurotransmitter after its release from the presynaptic nerve terminal. This is usually a catabolic enzyme system or an active reuptake mechanism.

112. The answer is E. *(Kaplan, 6/e, pp 144–153.)* Prospective longitudinal studies are studies in which persons who are "vulnerable" (i.e., at high risk for psychiatric illness because of a positive family history) are identified at birth and followed over a period of time. Such studies are less subject to methodological bias than other approaches. For example, when compared with retrospective studies, prospective longitudinal studies tend to give a more accurate representation of early signs and symptoms of a given disorder and thus offer a better opportunity for the discovery of successful preventive approaches.

113. The answer is C. *(Yudofsky, 2/e, pp 29–39.)* Information is transmitted along a neuron by way of a bioelectrical process that is partially dependent on properties of the cell membrane. These properties result in a voltage difference that is maintained across the membrane of an inactive neuron. Incoming stimuli depolarize the membrane, and if a threshold level is reached, an action potential is generated that reverses the polarity of the membrane. Propagation of the action potential down the axon, to its terminal button, causes the release of neurotransmitter into the synaptic cleft.

114. The answer is A. *(Kaplan, 6/e, p 1090. Yudofsky, 2/e, pp 7–13.)* Putative central nervous system neurotransmitters are generally classified in three groups: amino acids, biogenic amines, and neuropeptides. GABA is an inhibitory amino acid. The biogenic amines include the catecholamines (e.g., dopamine, norepinephrine, epinephrine), acetylcholine, histamine, and indolamines (e.g., serotonin). The neuropeptides include such substances as beta-endorphin, somatostatin, and vasopressin.

115. The answer is D. *(Kaplan, 6/e, p 82.)* REM sleep is often referred to as dream sleep. During REM sleep, blood pressure and heart rate tend to be variable, and penile tumescence is common. Decreased skeletal muscle tone always accompanies REM sleep.

116. The answer is E. *(Kaplan, 6/e, p 82.)* NREM sleep is commonly associated with decreased blood pressure and heart rate. Dreaming may occur but is infrequent, as are penile erections. Night terrors occur during NREM sleep, along with somnambulism and panic attacks.

117. The answer is A. *(Hales, 2/e, pp 537–538.)* Serotonin (5-hydroxytryptamine) has been implicated in the pathogenesis of obsessive-compulsive disorder (OCD). This has been supported by the antiobsessional effects of serotonin reuptake inhibitors. Noradrenergic antidepressants have not shown similar effectiveness.

118–121. The answers are 118-C, 119-A, 120-D, 121-B. *(Hales, 2/e, pp 13–27.)* CNS neurotransmitters include amino acids, biogenic amines, and neuropeptides. There are many other neurotransmitter substances, and many are still poorly understood. This is one of the most exciting areas of current psychiatric research. As more and more knowledge accrues, it becomes possible to develop more specific psychopharmacologic interventions. The amino acids are excitatory (glutamic acid, aspartic acid) or inhibitory (GABA). The biogenic amines include the catecholamines such as dopamine, norepinephrine, and epinephrine. Other biogenic amines include acetylcholine, histamine, and the indolamine serotonin. There are numerous neuropeptides, including beta-endorphin, somatostatin, and vasopressin.

122–126. The answers are 122-B, 123-C, 124-D, 125-A, 126-E. *(Kaplan, 6/e, pp 22–23.)* The hypothalamus plays a central role in regulating a variety of psychologic functions that directly affect behavior and thus is key to the biologic expression of psychiatric illness. Sleep, appetite, and sexual and aggressive behavior are subject to its control. In addition, the hypothalamus regulates temperature, fluid balance, and pituitary function.

Through electrical stimulation and ablation studies, hypothalamic nuclei have been identified as having defined functions. The anterior nucleus appears to facilitate sexual interest and specific sexual behavior; lesions in this area eliminate the behavior. The ventromedial nucleus acts as a satiety center; stimulation of this area reduces appetite. The ventromedial nucleus exerts its control through inhibition of the lateral nucleus, which stimulates appetite. Ablation of the lateral nucleus results in fatal anorexia regardless of the state of the ventromedial nucleus. The posterior nucleus along with the contiguous reticular activating system controls the level of arousal; lesions in this area result in lethargy and somnolence. Aggression appears to be affected by stimulation of a number of different hypothalamic sites.

The hypothalamus also exerts control over the pituitary gland. The supraoptic and paraventricular hypothalamic nuclei produce vasopressin (antidiuretic hormone) and oxytocin, respectively. These hormones traverse the axons of their parent neurons to the posterior pituitary gland, from which they are released. The hypothalamus also produces a variety of releasing factors that control hormone secretion from the anterior pituitary gland.

127–128. The answers are 127-C, 128-A. *(Hales, 2/e, pp 370–373.)* Many methods are used in the treatment of overdose. Ipecac to induce vomiting is commonly used with acetaminophen, salicylates, amphetamine, benzodiazepines, hypnotics, and phenothiazine, but not with alcohol or cocaine. Hemodialysis is commonly used with alcohol, amphetamine, and salicylates, but not with acetaminophen, cocaine, or tricyclics.

129–132. The answers are 129-C, 130-A, 131-D, 132-E. *(Hales, 2/e, pp 370–372. Isselbacher, 13/e, pp 1475, 2459.)* Each listed substance may be associated with multiple complications, though characterized by a major complication that is usually present. Cocaine overdose is particularly likely to be associated with seizures and acidosis along with psychological symptoms that often include agitation and psychotic symptoms. Phencyclidine is often recognized by the characteristic agitation, nystagmus, and hypertension. Other signs and symptoms may include agitation, aggressive behavior, muscle rigidity, and even hyperthermia and coma. The overdose symptoms of the tricyclic antidepressants are associated particularly with the anticholinergic effects of these drugs, with hypotension and cardiac side effects being prominent. In high overdosage, death may occur within 2 to 6 h following ingestion. Liver toxicity, peaking within 96 h, is a major medical problem associated with overdose with acetaminophen. It may lead to hepatic necrosis.

Disorders of Childhood and Adolescence

DIRECTIONS: Each item below contains a question or incomplete statement followed by suggested responses. Select the **one best** response to each question.

133. All the following drugs are commonly used by clinicians to treat the symptoms of attention-deficit hyperactivity disorder EXCEPT

(A) lorazepam
(B) amphetamine
(C) clonidine
(D) imipramine
(E) methylphenidate

134. The percentage of children with mental retardation who also exhibit attention-deficit hyperactivity disorder is approximately

(A) 0
(B) 1 to 2
(C) 10 to 20
(D) 40 to 50
(E) 70 to 80

135. The formation of core gender identity, one's biological self-designation as a male or female, is commonly believed to include all the following EXCEPT

(A) sex assignment at birth
(B) the neurophysiological organization of the fetal brain
(C) parental attitudes toward the child's sex
(D) the resolution of the oedipal conflict
(E) conditioning and other primitive forms of learning

136. All the following symptoms are commonly associated with the diagnosis of Tourette's disorder EXCEPT

(A) sleep disturbance
(B) obscene gestures
(C) echolalia
(D) obscene utterances
(E) hyperactivity and impulsiveness

137. The majority of mentally retarded persons are classified as mildly retarded, with IQs on standard psychological tests of

(A) below 34
(B) 35 to 49
(C) 50 to 70
(D) 71 to 85
(E) 85 to 95

138. Children diagnosed as having attention-deficit disorder, also called minimal brain dysfunction (MBD), would be LEAST likely to display which of the following signs?

(A) Impulsivity
(B) Social inappropriateness
(C) Hyperactivity
(D) Difficulty concentrating
(E) Severe neurologic deficits

139. An accurate characterization of mental retardation is that it is

(A) seen in 0.5 percent of the population
(B) more common in females
(C) more common in the upper social classes
(D) associated with progressive physical deterioration in Tay-Sachs disease
(E) diagnosed if the IQ is less than 90

140. Down's syndrome is correctly characterized by which of the following statements?

(A) It is most frequently a non-inherited chromosomal disorder
(B) It rarely involves trisomy
(C) It cannot be diagnosed antenatally
(D) It is a relatively rare cause of mental retardation
(E) It is most often associated with mild mental retardation

141. Childhood stuttering is most accurately described by which of the following statements?

(A) It is more common in girls than boys
(B) Affected children often outgrow the problem
(C) A family history of stuttering is rarely elicited
(D) It is very commonly associated with major mental illness
(E) Affected children usually have hysterical personality traits

142. True statements about autistic disorder include all the following EXCEPT

(A) it may be identifiable during the first 6 months of life
(B) it may manifest itself in resistance to minor environmental changes
(C) it is often associated with language disturbances
(D) it is rarely associated with mental retardation
(E) it is often associated with gaze aversion

143. All the following are commonly seen in infants with fetal alcohol syndrome EXCEPT

(A) normal intelligence
(B) microcephaly
(C) irritability
(D) midfacial hypoplasia and prognathism
(E) growth retardation

144. True statements about separation anxiety disorder include all the following EXCEPT

(A) it often runs in families
(B) it most commonly appears at puberty
(C) it is often associated with school absenteeism
(D) it is seen commonly in both boys and girls
(E) it is commonly seen in association with major depressive disorder

145. Correct statements about functional enuresis include that it

(A) has an onset prior to age 13
(B) most commonly occurs just prior to morning awakening
(C) is rarely if ever associated with daytime incontinence
(D) occurs more often in girls than boys
(E) is rarely associated with other emotional or behavioral symptoms

146. Characterize developmental reading disorder (dyslexia).

(A) It is diagnosed on the basis of a defect in visual or hearing acuity
(B) It is often associated with spelling and verbal language difficulties
(C) It occurs in less than 1 percent of the population
(D) It occurs more often in girls than boys
(E) It is often associated with brainstem neurologic defects

147. All the following statements about obsessive compulsive disorder (OCD) in early life are true EXCEPT

(A) it may occur as early as age 2
(B) the most common age of onset is adolescence
(C) symptoms are usually ego-dystonic in childhood
(D) the patient may be treated with clomipramine
(E) there is a family history of OCD in about 20 percent of these patients

148. Acute lead encephalopathy in children includes all the following EXCEPT

(A) irritability
(B) pallor
(C) vomiting
(D) seizures
(E) diarrhea

149. Schizophrenia that occurs in childhood

(A) has an earlier onset in boys than in girls
(B) is less common in boys than in girls when it occurs before the age of 12
(C) is significantly related to birth order
(D) generally has a more benign course than adult onset schizophrenia
(E) is usually associated with a very abnormal early developmental history

150. The pharmacological agent most commonly used by clinicians to treat primary nocturnal enuresis in children is

(A) clonazepam
(B) haloperidol
(C) phenytoin
(D) imipramine
(E) lithium

151. Suicide may be characterized by which of the following statements?

(A) It is a higher risk in girls than boys for children under the age of 12
(B) Attempts tend to be more serious in girls than in boys before puberty
(C) Attempts tend to be more lethal in girls than in boys during adolescence
(D) Attempts are more common in adolescent girls than in adolescent boys
(E) It is more often committed by adolescent girls than by adolescent boys

Disorders of Childhood and Adolescence

Answers

133. The answer is A. *(Schatzberg, pp 671–677.)* Stimulants were among the first drugs to be used as an effective psychopharmacologic treatment of attention-deficit hyperactivity disorder. Up to 80 percent of children have been reported to be improved with this treatment. Methylphenidate is believed by many clinicians to have the fewest side effects, and is often used as the drug of choice. Pemoline is used less often because of potential hypersensitivity reactions. Tricyclics have been reported to be effective, but cardiac arrhythmia may be a serious complication even at low dosage. Clonidine is useful in modulating mood and activity level, with little effect on attention. Benzodiazepines are not used in this condition.

134. The answer is C. *(Schatzberg, p 696.)* Approximately 10 to 20 percent of children with mental retardation will also exhibit attention-deficit hyperactivity disorder (ADHD). Mental retardation can also be associated with other mental disorders, such as schizophrenia and mood disorders. The children with ADHD show the same responsiveness to treatment as do nonretarded patients.

135. The answer is D. *(Nersessian, p 359.)* All the factors mentioned, with the exception of the oedipal conflict, were identified by R. Stoller in 1976 as factors that contribute to core gender identity, the conviction that one is male or female. This develops in the first 2 years of life, long before the developmental resolution of the oedipal conflict. Most clinicians believe that for most children gender assignment and rearing are more influential than anatomy.

136. The answer is A. *(Yudofsky, 2/e, pp 650–651.)* The typical findings in Tourette's disorder are multifocal motor and phonic tics. Tics are sudden, repetitive, and stereotyped motor movements that may be seen (e.g., eye blinking, jerking, gestures) or heard (e.g., throat clearing, coughing, echolalia, and obscene or "dirty" utterances). Motor hyperactivity and impulsiveness frequently precede the development of tics, and tics often begin as early as 5 years of age.

137. The answer is C. *(Hales, 2/e, pp 772–776.)* About 90 percent of persons with mental retardation test between 50 to 70 and are classified as mildly retarded. The commonly used tests are either the Stanford-Binet or the Wechsler. These children are often not distinguishable from other children until later in childhood and generally are able to learn academic skills up to approximately the sixth grade level. With proper social and vocational education they can generally live in the community and achieve minimum levels of self-support.

138. The answer is E. *(Yudofsky, 2/e, pp 646–648.)* Children with attention-deficit disorder generally display hyperactivity as their initial symptom, with an onset before age 7. Often at about age 10 the attentional symptoms become more important, and these children display impulsiveness, difficulty concentrating, easy distractibility, social inappropriateness, and poor judgment. Neurologic examination may be normal or show minimal nonspecific findings. Severe neurologic deficit is not generally found in this condition.

139. The answer is D. *(Andreasen, 2/e, pp 557–560.)* Mental retardation is more common in males. The male:female ratio is approximately 2:1. It is very common, affecting 1 to 2 percent of the population. While mild retardation is more common in the lower social classes, moderate and severe forms are equally common in all social classes. Some forms of mental retardation, such as Tay-Sachs disease, are characterized by severe and progressive physical deterioration and premature death.

140. The answer is A. *(Yudofsky, 2/e, pp 655–656.)* Down's syndrome is most frequently a noninherited chromosomal disorder that involves trisomy of the 21st chromosome. Many other cases are inherited, but clinically it is not possible to differentiate between the two forms of this disorder. Both forms can be diagnosed by chorionic villi sampling or by amniocentesis. Down's syndrome is the most commonly identified cause of mental retardation, and these patients are usually moderately to severely retarded.

141. The answer is B. *(Kaplan, 6/e, pp 2272–2275.)* The causes of stuttering are not known. While the incidence of stuttering in the relatives of affected persons is higher than that found in the general population, genetic factors are unclear. Boys are more commonly and chronically affected than are girls. No particular personality organization is typical, and there is no connection with major mental illness. It is estimated that about 40 percent or more of affected children ultimately outgrow the problem.

142. The answer is D. *(Yudofsky, 2/e, pp 644–645.)* Autistic disorder is a relatively uncommon but very severe disorder often associated with mental retardation. It may be clinically apparent early in infancy. Gaze aversion, which is not usually seen in normal development, is common. The disorder affects social, language, and imaginative development; most striking is the failure to develop typical social reciprocity with the mother and other caretakers. These patients are often ritualistic, preoccupied, and made uncomfortable by minor environmental changes.

143. The answer is A. *(Yudofsky, 2/e, pp 652–653.)* The classical findings in fetal alcoholism include mild to moderate mental retardation, which is reported in up to 85 percent of the cases. The mechanism of the teratogenic effects is not well understood, but these effects include microcephaly, irritability, intrauterine and postnatal growth retardation, midfacial hypoplasia, and prognathism. The complete picture is seen in about 1 to 2 live births per 1000, but partial expression may occur in as many as 5 live births per 1000.

144. The answer is B. *(Kaplan, 6/e, pp 2345–2348.)* Separation anxiety disorder is common, and the usual onset is in early to mid-childhood. It is commonly associated with school absenteeism and can precede or be associated with major depression in children. It occurs in both boys and girls, seems to run in families, and tends to be a chronic condition.

145. The answer is B. *(Kaplan, 6/e, pp 2337–2340.)* Functional enuresis may occur in both the daytime and nighttime and more commonly has an onset in childhood, with the incidence in boys being somewhat higher. Adolescent onsets do occur and tend to be associated with more psychopathology and to have a poorer prognosis. Nocturnal enuresis usually occurs 30 min to 3 h after the onset of sleep. About half of enuretic children have other associated emotional disturbances, though it is sometimes difficult to separate cause and effect.

146. The answer is B. *(Kaplan, 6/e, pp 2246–2250.)* Dyslexia occurs in 3 to 10 percent of the population and is more often found in boys than in girls. When a reading disorder is caused by a defect in visual or hearing acuity, it is excluded by diagnostic criteria from the diagnosis of developmental reading disorder. Almost all patients with this problem have spelling difficulties, and nearly all have verbal language defects. It is believed that the most common etiology relates to cortical brain pathology.

147. The answer is C. *(Yudofsky, 2/e, pp 648–650.)* OCD has been diagnosed as early as 2 years of age, but there appears to be an increased incidence at age 7 and in late adolescence. About 20 percent of these patients have a positive family history for OCD in a first-degree relative. The ego-dystonia of obsessions or compulsions that characterizes adolescent or adult onset is often absent in patients who develop the disorder during childhood. Patients are often treated with clomipramine.

148. The answer is E. *(Yudofsky, 2/e, p 653.)* Acute lead encephalopathy is seen less frequently than in the past, but when it occurs, the prodromal symptoms include pallor, vomiting, irritability, sometimes weight loss, and constipation, which serves to increase absorption. Overt symptoms can include seizure activity, cranial nerve palsy, and ataxia. Increased intracranial pressure may ensue, and death occurs in about one-quarter of these patients.

149. The answer is A. *(Kaplan, 6/e, pp 2393–2398.)* Onset of schizophrenia is rare prior to puberty, but when it occurs, it is among the most severe of all psychiatric disorders. While adult schizophrenia is equally common in males and females, childhood onset is more common in males than females, and males usually have an earlier age of onset. Occurrence is unrelated to birth order, and many or most of these children have an unremarkable early developmental history, though a delay in language acquisition is relatively common.

150. The answer is D. *(Schatzberg, pp 694–695.)* Low doses of tricyclic antidepressants, most commonly imipramine, are commonly used to treat primary nocturnal enuresis. The mechanism of action is unclear, but does not seem to be related to the alteration of sleep architecture. Though more expensive, desmopressin acetate (DDAVP), an analogue of antidiuretic hormone, is also effective.

151. The answer is D. *(Kaplan, 6/e, pp 2384–2391.)* Patterns of suicide and suicide attempts show definite gender differences in both childhood and adolescence. In childhood boys are more likely to develop suicidal behavior, but there is no significant gender difference in the seriousness of suicide attempts. In contrast, adolescent girls are more likely than boys to attempt suicide, but the attempts by boys are more lethal and more often successful.

Cognitive Disorders and Consultation-Liaison Psychiatry

DIRECTIONS: Each item below contains a question or incomplete statement followed by suggested responses. Select the **one best** response to each question.

152. The syndrome of delirium is characterized by all the following EXCEPT

(A) depressed affect
(B) inattention
(C) disorientation and confusion
(D) global cognitive changes
(E) perceptual disturbances

153. Cluster headaches are characterized by all the following EXCEPT

(A) they have no known precipitants
(B) they are more common in females
(C) they are sometimes associated with agitation and head banging
(D) they usually occur in series
(E) they generally consist of severe, unilateral pain

154. The onset of primary dementia of the Alzheimer type is

(A) abrupt
(B) most common after the age of 65
(C) associated only with memory changes
(D) secondary to medical illness
(E) unaccompanied by changes in personality and behavior

155. Pick's disease is characterized by all the following EXCEPT

(A) it accounts for about 5 percent of the irreversible dementias
(B) it is clinically indistinguishable from Alzheimer's disease
(C) it can be definitively diagnosed only after death
(D) it is associated with frontotemporal atrophy and ventricular dilatation
(E) it is more common in women

156. All the following statements about complex partial seizures are true EXCEPT

(A) they are one variety of temporal lobe seizures
(B) impaired consciousness or loss of contact with the environment occurs
(C) the patient remembers associated automatisms as uncontrollable events
(D) associated automatisms can be ictal or postictal
(E) the focus is in temporal (limbic) structures

157. All the following symptoms are commonly associated with premenstrual syndrome (PMS) EXCEPT

(A) anxiety
(B) irritability
(C) elation
(D) tension
(E) depression

158. Clinical observations of emotional responses in the premenstruum show which of the following?

(A) Girls tend to repeat the symptom patterns of their mothers
(B) Symptoms cease when daughters leave their parental home
(C) About 50 percent of women experience severe symptoms
(D) Symptoms tend to peak in the second decade of life
(E) None of the above

159. Normal pressure hydrocephalus is usually associated with dementia, gait disturbance, and

(A) urinary incontinence
(B) seizures
(C) visual hallucinations
(D) auditory hallucinations
(E) aphasia

160. All the following statements about absence seizures are true EXCEPT

(A) they are also known as petit mal
(B) they are associated with an abrupt loss of attention to the environment
(C) the patient does not usually show confusion following the episode
(D) the loss of consciousness is usually for between 1 and 2 min
(E) during a seizure the patient may stare blankly or show automatisms such as lip smacking

161. Correct statements about chronic subdural hematomas include all the following EXCEPT

(A) the majority are caused by head injury
(B) the most common symptom is headache
(C) the symptoms may progress over days to weeks
(D) fluctuations of consciousness often occur
(E) focal or lateralizing signs are rarely if ever present

162. Temporal lobe epilepsy has been associated with all the following personality characteristics EXCEPT

(A) obsessiveness
(B) hypersexuality
(C) mood variability
(D) hyperreligiosity
(E) paranoid ideation

163. The occurrence of delusions de novo in a person over the age of 35 years, and without a known history of schizophrenia or delusional disorder, should always alert the diagnostician to the possibility of

(A) agoraphobia
(B) frotteurism
(C) sleep disorder
(D) substance abuse
(E) dissociative disorder

164. Psychiatric features commonly found in patients with Addison's disease include all the following EXCEPT

(A) depression
(B) memory impairment
(C) irritability
(D) excessive energy
(E) anxiety

165. Huntington's disease is associated with all the following EXCEPT

(A) autosomal dominant inheritance
(B) acute onset
(C) onset during adulthood
(D) personality changes
(E) cerebral atrophy

166. In which of the following age groups is the incidence of psychopathology the greatest?

(A) Under 10 years
(B) 10 to 25 years
(C) 25 to 45 years
(D) 45 to 65 years
(E) Over 65 years

Items 167–169

A 22-year-old woman is admitted to the hospital because of right-hand anesthesia that developed after an argument with her brother. She is in good spirits and seems unconcerned about her problem. There is no history of physical trauma. The neurologic examination is negative except for reduced sensitivity to pain in a glove-like distribution over the right hand. Her entire family is in attendance and is expressing great concern and attentiveness. She ignores her brother and seems unaware of the chronic jealousy and rivalry described by her family.

167. The most likely diagnosis is

(A) body dysmorphic disorder
(B) histrionic personality disorder
(C) parietal brain tumor
(D) conversion disorder
(E) hysteria

168. The absence of anxiety in association with her lack of awareness of the psychological conflict with her brother is most likely due to

(A) marginal intellectual function
(B) hypochondriasis
(C) organic mental dysfunction
(D) primary gain
(E) psychosis

169. The patient's seeming enjoyment of the attention and concern of her family is most likely due to

(A) primary gain
(B) secondary gain
(C) tertiary gain
(D) indifference reaction
(E) suppression

170. The most common cause of hyperprolactinemia in the psychiatric patient is

(A) neuroleptic medication
(B) oral contraceptives
(C) hypothyroidism
(D) cirrhosis
(E) pregnancy

171. All the following psychoactive drugs should be avoided in patients with porphyria EXCEPT

(A) chlorpromazine
(B) carbamazepine
(C) phenobarbital
(D) cocaine
(E) chlordiazepoxide

172. A man given a placebo for mild pain reports 30 min later that the pain has resolved. The most appropriate conclusion is that the man

(A) has a conversion disorder
(B) has a dissociative disorder
(C) is malingering
(D) had no real pain to begin with
(E) responds to placebos

173. A 62-year-old woman is admitted to a medical unit because of an 11.4-kg (25-lb) weight loss over the last 3 months. She also reports anorexia, insomnia, fatigue, and decreased sexual interest. She does not have depressed affect, and her mental status is judged to be unimpaired. Extensive medical evaluation is unremarkable. The most likely diagnosis is

(A) senile dementia
(B) occult malignancy
(C) hypochondriasis
(D) chronic anxiety
(E) masked depression

174. All the following medical conditions may result in depression secondary to hypercalcemia EXCEPT

(A) ingestion of excess vitamin D
(B) multiple myeloma
(C) renal tumors
(D) general paresis
(E) Paget's disease

175. Multi-infarct dementia is

(A) an extremely rare form of dementia
(B) characterized by rapid onset
(C) usually seen after the age of 75
(D) not associated with neurological impairment
(E) rarely associated with hypertension

176. The most common cause of dementia in the elderly is

(A) multiple cerebral infarcts
(B) normal pressure hydrocephalus
(C) Alzheimer's disease
(D) Huntington's disease
(E) hardening of cerebral arteries

177. The sudden loss of muscular strength in association with laughter is most consistent with which of the following conditions?

(A) Catatonia
(B) Epilepsy
(C) Cataplexy
(D) Narcolepsy
(E) Hysteria

178. Symptoms of hyperventilation syndrome commonly include all the following EXCEPT

(A) perioral tingling
(B) carpopedal spasm
(C) fainting
(D) inappropriate laughter or crying
(E) visual hallucinations

179. Symptoms that commonly occur in patients presenting with AIDS-dementia complex include all the following EXCEPT

(A) focal seizure activity
(B) cognitive abnormalities
(C) motor abnormalities
(D) behavioral abnormalities
(E) mood abnormalities

180. Cognitive disorders typically are characterized by

(A) mental confusion, disorientation, and memory loss
(B) mental confusion, auditory hallucinations, and thought disorder
(C) depression, auditory hallucinations, and disorientation
(D) depression, visual hallucinations, and thought disorder
(E) depression, grandiosity, and sleep disorder

181. All the following statements about the condition known as obstructive sleep apnea are true EXCEPT that it is

(A) more common in men than in women
(B) more common in middle-aged adults than in children
(C) associated with excessive daytime hypervigilance
(D) often associated with snoring
(E) often associated with hypertension

182. The odor of garlic on the breath occurs soon after acute poisoning with

(A) thallium
(B) lead
(C) arsenic
(D) aluminum
(E) manganese

183. Olfactory hallucinations are relatively rare and are most commonly encountered in patients with

(A) parietal tumors
(B) narcolepsy
(C) grand mal epilepsy
(D) partial complex seizures
(E) Wilson's disease

184. The most common psychiatric disturbance associated with Cushing's syndrome is

(A) depression
(B) psychosis
(C) organic mental disorder
(D) mania
(E) anxiety neurosis

185. All the following are commonly found in normal pressure hydrocephalus EXCEPT

(A) incontinence
(B) dementia
(C) gait disturbance
(D) apathy
(E) aphasia

186. True statements about post-cardiac surgery delirium include all the following EXCEPT

(A) it is the most common psychiatric complication of cardiac surgery
(B) it most commonly develops 2 to 4 days after surgery
(C) it is more common in dominant as opposed to dependent personalities
(D) it is more common in patients who express high preoperative anxiety
(E) It is more common in patients with a history of myocardial infarction

Items 187–190

A 55-year-old man presents with the chief complaint of feelings of helplessness, hopelessness, loss of interest, and poor sleep for the past 3 weeks. He is about 25 pounds overweight, smokes a pack of cigarettes a day, and has multiple physical complaints. He was fired from his job of 20 years 6 weeks ago. One month ago it was discovered that he has hypertension, and he was started on antihypertensive medication.

187. The patient's differential diagnosis should include all the following EXCEPT

(A) dysthymia
(B) adjustment disorder with depressed mood
(C) major depressive disorder
(D) mood disorder due to medical condition or treatment
(E) substance abuse

188. If this patient began complaining of impotence for the first time, the most likely cause would be

(A) disorder of core gender identity
(B) drug effect
(C) primary impotence
(D) penile steal syndrome
(E) dementia

189. If psychopharmacological intervention was prescribed for his symptoms, the most likely medication would be

(A) fluoxetine
(B) phenobarbital
(C) lithium
(D) buspirone
(E) phenytoin

190. It is unlikely that the patient's mood changes are secondary to schizophrenia, which is characterized by all the following EXCEPT

(A) the dysphoric mood is usually apathetic or empty
(B) there is a more gradual onset
(C) hallucinations and delusions are constant
(D) there is often more deterioration of general functioning
(E) psychotic symptoms tend to persist after mood symptoms remit

191. Elisabeth Kübler-Ross has described five major phases that occur in a person's psychological adjustment to impending death. These include all the following EXCEPT

(A) acceptance
(B) denial
(C) anger
(D) theorizing
(E) bargaining

192. Tertiary prevention refers to

(A) forestalling the recurrence of psychiatric symptoms
(B) psychopharmacologic intervention during remission
(C) treatment of current manifest symptoms
(D) anticipating and preventing the development of psychiatric symptoms
(E) use of paraprofessionals

193. The orbitofrontal syndrome sometimes seen in neoplasms of the frontal lobe is characterized by all the following EXCEPT

(A) disinhibition
(B) impulsivity
(C) poor insight
(D) emotional blandness
(E) poor judgment

DIRECTIONS: Each group of questions below consists of lettered options followed by numbered items. For each numbered item, select the appropriate lettered option(s). Each lettered option may be used once, more than once, or not at all. **Choose exactly the number of options indicated following each item.**

Items 194–197

Match each description with the appropriate disorder.

(A) Wernicke's encephalopathy
(B) Korsakoff's psychosis
(C) Huntington's disease
(D) Wilson's disease
(E) Creutzfeldt-Jakob disease

194. Rapidly progressive and fatal dementia with a usual age of onset in the forties or fifties. **(SELECT 1 DISORDER)**

195. An abrupt onset with oculomotor disturbances, cerebellar ataxia, and mental confusion. **(SELECT 1 DISORDER)**

196. A chronic condition that characteristically presents with confabulation and memory problems. **(SELECT 1 DISORDER)**

197. A disorder characterized by choreiform movements and dementia, with an age of onset usually in the thirties. **(SELECT 1 DISORDER)**

Items 198–204

Match each concept with the correct name.

(A) Elisabeth Kübler-Ross
(B) Franz Alexander
(C) Sigmund Freud
(D) Wilhelm Reich
(E) Flanders Dunbar

198. Psychosomatic illnesses are associated with specific unresolved neurotic conflicts. **(SELECT 1 NAME)**

199. There are seven psychosomatic illnesses: bronchial asthma, ulcerative colitis, rheumatoid arthritis, essential hypertension, peptic ulcer disease, neurodermatitis, and Graves' disease. **(SELECT 1 NAME)**

200. Hysterical neurosis results from memories that have been repressed. **(SELECT 1 NAME)**

201. Psychosomatic illnesses are characterized by specific personality traits. **(SELECT 1 NAME)**

202. Persons experiencing life-threatening illness go through distinct stages of psychological adjustment. **(SELECT 1 NAME)**

203. Psychoanalysis should address the underlying character type as well as symptoms. **(SELECT 1 NAME)**

204. Hysterical (i.e., histrionic) personality is characterized by seductiveness, excitability, and superficial interpersonal relationships. **(SELECT 1 NAME)**

Cognitive Disorders and Consultation-Liaison Psychiatry

Answers

152. The answer is A. *(Andreasen, 2/e, pp 178–181.)* Delirious states usually have a sudden onset, often in the context of a medical illness. The most common finding is a defect in attention, global cognitive impairment, and disorientation and confusion. The patient is often unable to complete a coherent sentence and may misperceive distracting stimuli. Disturbance of consciousness may extend from quietness and a tendency to fall asleep all the way to lethargy, stupor, or coma. Some patients display hypervigilance or agitation or have illusions or hallucinations.

153. The answer is B. *(Kaplan, 6/e, pp 254–255.)* Cluster headache is relatively uncommon. It occurs five to six times more commonly in males. The attacks usually consist of constant and severe, stabbing, unilateral pain that lasts 15 min to 3 h. The attacks usually occur in series. The pathophysiology is unknown.

154. The answer is B. *(Andreasen, 2/e, pp 187–190.)* Alzheimer's disease is the most common of the degenerative dementias. The late onset variety, occurring at age 65 or older, is the most common. In addition to memory impairment, aphasia, apraxia, or agnosia is often present. The course is characterized by gradual onset and continuing cognitive decline.

155. The answer is E. *(Andreasen, 2/e, p 190.)* Pick's disease accounts for about 5 percent of the irreversible dementias, and the clinical presentation is often identical to Alzheimer's dementia. Autopsy examination is necessary for the diagnosis and discloses the distinctive frontotemporal atrophy and ventricular dilatation, along with gliosis and Pick's bodies in the neurons. Pick's disease is more common in men and first-degree relatives.

156. The answer is C. *(Yudofsky, 2/e, p 401.)* Impairment of consciousness is a hallmark of complex partial seizures. The focal discharge is associated with a temporal aura, and as this discharge spreads to the limbic system, impaired consciousness and loss of contact with the environment ensue. Automatisms are highly integrated, unconscious movements not remembered by the patient. They commonly include such activities as lip smacking, rubbing, running, disrobing, or the perseveration of acts initiated prior to loss of consciousness. Automatisms can be ictal or postictal events.

157. The answer is C. *(Kaplan, 6/e, pp 110–111, 1698.)* A wide variety of emotional and physical symptoms have been associated with premenstrual syndrome. These include irritability, anxiety, depression, and generalized tension. Elation is not generally reported. Physical symptoms include breast tenderness, abdominal bloating, and swelling of the ankles.

158. The answer is A. *(Rundell, pp 722–725.)* Clinical observations and study of menstrual responses in families have shown a tendency for girls to repeat the symptom patterns of their mothers. These do not change when the daughter leaves home. About 5 to 10 percent of women in the United States have severe menstrual symptoms, and these tend to peak in the fourth decade of life.

159. The answer is A. *(Yudofsky, 2/e, p 614.)* Many dementias are chronic, slowly progressive, and unresponsive to treatment. One major exception is normal-pressure hydrocephalus. It is difficult to diagnose, but often is precipitated by such acute events as trauma, subarachnoid hemorrhage, or meningitis. Classically it is associated with gait ataxia and urinary incontinence. Headaches and papilledema are absent. Clinical improvement is sometimes dramatic when the cerebrospinal fluid is shunted away from the central nervous system into the cardiovascular system.

160. The answer is D. *(Yudofsky, 2/e, p 400.)* During an absence seizure, also called petit mal, the patient has an abrupt loss of attention while remaining awake and maintaining posture. The seizure activity rarely lasts beyond 20 s, and the patient displays an abrupt return of attention without residual confusion. Stereotyped or automatic behavior (such as lip smacking, chewing, or blinking) is common, but there is not a generalized convulsion. Some patients may show mild clonic, atonic, or tonic activity.

161. The answer is E. *(Isselbacher, 13/e, pp 144, 2323. Yudofsky, 2/e, p 454.)* The majority (about 60 percent) of chronic subdural hematomas follow head trauma. Other causes include ruptured aneurysms and rapid deceleration injuries to the brain. Headache is the most common symptom. As intracranial pressure gradually increases, signs associated with dementia appear including apathy, memory loss, drowsiness, and ultimately coma. Fluctuations in the level of consciousness predominate over focal or lateralizing neurologic signs, though such signs are not rare.

162. The answer is B. *(Yudofsky, 2/e, p 237.)* While the issue of personality change caused by partial complex seizures (temporal lobe seizures) is an area of some controversy, many investigators believe there is a common constellation of personality symptoms. These include obsessiveness, elaborated conversation, mood variability, hyperreligiosity, hypergraphia, irritability, and paranoia. Typically these patients are hyposexual rather than hypersexual.

163. The answer is D. *(DSM-IV, pp 281–285.)* Schizophrenia and delusional disorder often, but not always, first appear in persons under the age of 35 years. When delusions appear de novo without such a history, one must always consider the possibility of an organic delusional disorder. Abuses of substances such as cannabis, cocaine, amphetamines, and hallucinogens are common causes of organic delusional syndrome. Other causes include cerebral lesions and interictal phenomena in temporal lobe epilepsy.

164. The answer is D. *(Isselbacher, 13/e, pp 1970-1972.)* Psychiatric symptoms are very common in patients with Addison's disease, with estimates as high as 90 percent. Symptoms are quite varied and often insidious. Early on they include apathy, irritability, social withdrawal, negativism, and fatigue. In addition, many patients experience depression. Cognitive impairment, especially of memory, may be present and mental changes tend to be episodic. Excessive energy is not present.

165. The answer is B. *(Yudofsky, 2/e, pp 586–592.)* Huntington's disease is a rare illness that is inherited as an autosomal dominant trait and typically manifests during adulthood. It is characterized clinically by the insidious onset of choreïform movements, dementia, and personality changes. No effective treatment is presently known. At autopsy, the brain of affected persons is atrophied, especially in the caudate nucleus and putamen.

166. The answer is E. *(Kaplan, 6/e, pp 360–361.)* Persons older than 65 years of age have a higher risk than other persons of developing mental illness. However, elderly persons are underrepresented in the frequency of visits to mental health clinics and in the receipt of appropriate social services. Common psychiatric problems in this population include depression and organic mental disorders.

167–169. The answers are 167-D, 168-D, 169-B. *(Rundell, pp 387–390.)* This patient displays some of the classic findings in conversion disorder. She has an alteration of physical functioning that suggests a physical disorder, the altered function was precipitated by a psychological event, the pattern (glove-like anesthesia) cannot readily be explained by a known disorder, and physical findings are negative. Patients with body dysmorphic disorder are preoccupied with imagined defects in their appearance, which is normal. The term hysteria is used pejoratively to mean that the symptoms are not real, but it is not an actual diagnosis. Patients with a parietal tumor would likely have other signs and symptoms.

The patient's lack of anxiety and awareness of the existence and significance of the conflict with her brother is a classic finding in conversion disorder. It is an example of "primary gain." This refers to keeping an internal conflict or need out of awareness, reducing the anxiety associated with it, and finding a partial solution to the underlying conflict. The enjoyment of attention from her family is an example of "secondary gain," which serves to reinforce the symptom. There is no such thing as "tertiary gain," and suppression refers to placing something into the preconscious rather than the unconscious. The indifference reaction is associated with right hemispheric lesions and consists of symptoms of indifference toward failures, lack of interest in family and friends, enjoyment of foolish jokes, and minimizing physical difficulties.

170. The answer is A. *(Yudofsky, 2/e, pp 537–538.)* Even small doses of neuroleptic medication can produce hyperprolactinemia, and this is the most common etiology found in psychiatric patients. Other causes include severe systemic illness such as cirrhosis or renal failure, pregnancy, stress, neoplasm, and oral contraceptives. Hyperprolactinemia due to tumors is much more common in women than in men.

171. The answer is A. *(Isselbacher, 13/e, pp 407, 2076.)* There are a number of nonpsychiatric medications and psychoactive drugs that should not be used in patients with porphyria because of the danger of precipitating an acute episode. These include alcohol, oral contraceptives, phenytoin, barbiturates, sulfonamides, and valproic acid.

172. The answer is E. *(Rundell, p 1008.)* The only conclusion that can be reached about the man described in the question is that he responds to placebos. His response says nothing about whether his pain is "real" or psychogenic. Placebos have been shown to decrease pain of both psychological and physiologic origin.

173. The answer is E. *(Rundell, pp 316–321.)* Depressive illness consists of both somatic and psychological components. The somatic components include insomnia, anorexia, weight loss, fatigue, motor retardation or agitation, and decreased sexual interest. The psychological components include depressed mood, pessimism, and feelings of worthlessness and guilt. Not all components are present in every case. Patients who have a masked depression present with primarily somatic symptoms and few or no psychological ones. Diagnosis often is made only after extensive medical evaluation is unrevealing. The woman described in the question did not have any signs of dementia; medical evaluation did not reveal an organic disease process; and although hypochondriasis and chronic anxiety could have caused many of her symptoms, they are not likely to have caused the 11.4-kg weight loss.

174. The answer is D. *(Rundell, p 328.)* There are a number of metabolic diseases, including those secondary to vitamin excess or deficiency, that may result in mood disorders. All the listed diagnoses, except general paresis, can be associated with hypercalcemia of nonendocrine origin and can result in an anhedonic retarded depression. General paresis is most often associated with manic symptoms, but this is commonly followed by depression and then dementia.

175. The answer is B. *(Andreasen, 2/e, p 192.)* Multi-infarct dementia is the second most common cause of dementia. It is characterized by a rapid onset and a step-wise deterioration. It most commonly occurs in patients in their fifties or sixties and is often associated with hypertension or diabetes. Focal neurological impairment is common.

176. The answer is C. *(Andreasen, 2/e, pp 187–190.)* Although estimates vary, it is currently believed that 50 percent of demented elderly suffer from senile dementia of the Alzheimer type. The cause of this disorder is unknown, and no treatment for it exists. Approximately 20 percent of demented elderly suffer from cerebral arteriosclerosis (previously described as hardening of the cerebral arteries). Cerebral arteriosclerosis produces dementia by causing multiple cerebral infarcts. Normal pressure hydrocephalus and Huntington's disease are rare causes of dementia.

177. The answer is C. *(Andreasen, 2/e, p 603.)* Cataplexy is the sudden and brief loss of muscular tone that occurs during the expression of a strong emotion. Affected persons remain conscious throughout each episode, which usually lasts no longer than 2 min. Cataplexy often occurs in patients with narcolepsy who may also have hypnagogic phenomena and sleep paralysis. The cause is unknown.

178. The answer is E. *(Hales, 2/e, p 500.)* Hyperventilation occurs when there is increased respiration beyond that needed to maintain normal blood gases, and the resultant "blowing off" of carbon dioxide leads to respiratory alkalosis. The most common cause is anxiety. Symptoms may include tingling, carpopedal spasm or tetany, feelings of depersonalization or derealization, mood lability, and inappropriate crying or laughter. Hallucinations are not a part of the clinical picture.

179. The answer is A. *(Rundell, pp 824–825.)* Patients with AIDS-dementia complex generally have an insidious onset of the condition with a variety of mood, motor, cognitive, and behavioral symptoms. These include increasing difficulty with attention and memory, weakness, loss of balance, incoordination, apathy, depression, and withdrawal. Occasionally affective psychosis will occur. Such symptoms may be the first presentation of the HIV infection.

180. The answer is A. *(Rundell, pp 67–68.)* An organic mental disorder is characterized by disorientation, memory loss, mental confusion, and occasionally by visual hallucinations. The disorder occurs commonly in both medical and surgical patients and is often the result of metabolic abnormalities or adverse reactions to medication. When the disorder has an acute onset, reversible causes should be sought.

181. The answer is C. *(Rundell, pp 515–516.)* Sleep-disordered breathing is an important cause of persistent insomnia. It is more common in men than in women. The syndrome of obstructive sleep apnea is associated with excessive daytime sleepiness (not hypervigilance) and is often found in middle-aged, hypertensive, and overweight men. The bed partners of these patients complain bitterly about the patients' snoring.

182. The answer is C. *(Yudofsky, 2/e, pp 547–548.)* Acute arsenic poisoning may occur by accidental, suicidal, or homicidal ingestion. Within 30 min to 2 h the initial symptoms of garlic breath and a metallic taste will occur. This is followed by gastrointestinal inflammation, circulatory collapse, and CNS symptoms, which may include headache, vertigo, stupor, delirium, convulsions, and coma.

183. The answer is D. *(Yudofsky, 2/e, p 239.)* Hallucinations involving smell, taste, or kinesthetic experiences are rare. They are most commonly encountered in patients with partial complex seizures. They are also found at times in other organic or psychiatric disorders such as somatization disorder, psychosis, and hypochondriasis. Tumors involving the olfactory areas of the brain must also be considered.

184. The answer is A. *(Isselbacher, 13/e, pp 1960–1965.)* Cushing's syndrome often is associated with psychiatric disturbances. Depression is the most common disturbance and may range from moderate to severe; as many as 10 percent of affected persons attempt suicide. Mania, psychosis, and an organic mental disorder also can occur.

185. The answer is E. *(Yudofsky, 2/e, pp 614–615.)* The classic syndrome of normal pressure hydrocephalus consists of dementia, incontinence, and gait disturbance. The dementia frequently involves impaired attention, poor learning, and impaired abstraction and judgment. The syndrome does not commonly include aphasia, apraxia, or agnosia. These patients may have a variety of psychiatric symptoms, including anxiety, personality changes, and disturbance of mood.

186. The answer is D. *(Rundell, pp 617–623.)* Postcardiac surgery delirium is the most common psychiatric complication of cardiac surgery. While it may occur immediately, more commonly it follows a lucid period of 2 to 4 days. Patients with dominant personalities appear more likely to develop delirium, as do patients with low preoperative anxiety. This is probably due to difficulty in accepting the dependent sick role, while the denial of anxiety serves as an ineffective defense mechanism. Patients with a history of myocardial infarction are at higher risk probably because of cerebral anoxia secondary to diminished cardiac output.

187–190. The answers are 187-A, 188-B, 189-A, 190-C. *(Andreasen, 2/e, pp 247–288.)* In assessing this patient's presenting symptoms, the presence of a significant stressor (job loss) would necessitate consideration of an adjustment disorder. The presence of dysphoria lasting more than 2 weeks and associated with weight loss, sleep disturbance, decreased libido, and loss of interest necessitates consideration of a major depression. His depression might also be secondary to medication or to undeclared substance abuse. Dysthymia is not a consideration, since the diagnosis requires a depressed mood for at least 2 years.

In the absence of a previous history of impotence, the most likely cause of his current difficulty is either the hypertension medication or the direct effects of his depression. Both are frequent causes of impotence. A core gender identity disturbance would have been manifest since childhood.

Fluoxetine is a selective serotonin reuptake inhibitor (SSRI), a common first choice among available antidepressants. Lithium is used for both mania and depression but is not often the first medication selected in the absence of an indication of bipolar disorder. The other listed medications are not used for the primary treatment of depression.

The differential diagnosis of major depression and depressed mood associated with schizophrenia can be very difficult. In schizophrenia, the onset is usually more gradual. The mood is usually apathetic or empty, in comparison with the painful depressed mood that is more common to major depression. Both diagnoses can be associated with psychosis, but in schizophrenia, the mood disturbance tends to persist even after the psychosis has long disappeared.

191. The answer is D. *(Kaplan, 6/e, p 1715.)* Elisabeth Kübler-Ross has described five phases of psychological adjustment that people pass through when confronted with the knowledge that they are dying. Characteristically, the first stage involves denial of death and isolation of feelings. Affected persons then experience anger at their fate and may begin bargaining (often with God) to avert death. A period of depression finally is followed by acceptance. These responses do not necessarily occur in this sequence; several may occur simultaneously, or they may be mixed with other responses.

192. The answer is A. *(Rundell, p 43.)* In 1964, C. Caplan developed a model of psychiatric prevention. Primary prevention referred to anticipating and preventing the development of symptoms, primarily through early intervention. Secondary prevention referred to treating psychiatric symptoms when they are manifest. In tertiary prevention, the psychiatrist seeks to alter the sequelae that may follow an acute illness and acts to prevent recurrence of the illness.

193. The answer is D. *(Rundell, p 700.)* Neoplasms of the frontal lobe are likely to display psychiatric symptoms as much as 90 percent of the time. There are three potential types of dysfunction, one of which is the orbitofrontal syndrome. It is characterized by emotional disinhibition, impulsivity, poor insight, and poor judgment. Typically there is emotional lability with inappropriate jocularity and euphoria.

194–197. The answers are 194-E, 195-A, 196-B, 197-C. *(Yudofsky, 2/e, pp 573–574, 587–588, 599–600.)* Both Wernicke's and Korsakoff's syndromes are associated with thiamine deficiency, which often results from alcoholism. Wernicke's encephalopathy has an abrupt onset with mental confusion, cerebellar ataxia, and oculomotor disturbances such as nystagmus or gaze palsy. The general confusional state may ultimately worsen with the development of Korsakoff's psychosis and ultimately stupor and coma. Korsakoff's psychosis is chronic, with both retrograde and anterograde amnesia. Confabulation is common.

Creutzfeldt-Jakob disease may present with neurotic-like symptoms or as dementia and is fatal. It usually begins in the forties or fifties and rapidly progresses to severe dementia and death often in 1 year. It appears to be caused by a "slow" virus.

Wilson's disease is due to an inborn error of copper metabolism and usually has an onset in adolescence. The early onset with bizarre behavior and flattened affect may lead to a misdiagnosis of schizophrenia, although the neurologic signs usually precede the psychiatric symptoms. Not all cases show significant psychiatric symptoms.

Huntington's disease is a hereditary disorder that usually begins when the patient is in his or her late thirties. It is associated with choreiform movements and a progressive dementia that eventually, over decades, culminates in apathy and death.

198–204. The answers are 198-B, 199-B, 200-C, 201-E, 202-A, 203-D, 204-D. *(Kaplan, 6/e, pp 1463–1472.)* Sigmund Freud developed the concepts of psychological conflict and repression. He believed that persons who had hysterical neuroses suffered from the repression of memories and the feelings associated with them. His original ideas led to the development of psychoanalysis and laid the groundwork for psychosomatic medicine. Freud's early work was concerned mainly with symptoms.

Wilhelm Reich, a student of Freud, called attention to the importance of character types in diagnosis and treatment. One of the personality types he discussed was the hysterical personality, which he characterized as seductive, easily excitable, and superficial in interpersonal relationships.

Personality type and psychological conflict both have been cited as pathogenetic factors that cause physical symptoms and psychosomatic illnesses. Flanders Dunbar thought that persons who had psychosomatic illnesses had specific personality traits. Franz Alexander gave major impetus to the concept that the seven classic psychosomatic illnesses—bronchial asthma, ulcerative colitis, rheumatoid arthritis, essential hypertension, peptic ulcer disease, neurodermatitis, and Graves' disease—were characterized by specific, unresolved neurotic conflicts. For example, he felt that persons with peptic ulcer disease had conflicts about oral dependency. Recent investigators, however, have questioned the specificity of his formulations, in part because many neurotic conflicts occur in association with more illnesses than the seven listed by Alexander. In fact, most—if not all—medical and surgical illnesses have concomitant psychological factors; in that sense, they are all psychosomatic in nature.

Elisabeth Kübler-Ross has written extensively on psychological adjustment to impending death.

Schizophrenia and Other Psychotic Disorders

DIRECTIONS: Each item below contains a question or incomplete statement followed by suggested responses. Select the **one best** response to each question.

Items 205–208

A 25-year-old college student is admitted to a psychiatric ward with a history of "personality change, strange behavior, and weird ideas" for 6 months, and bizarre paranoid delusions and hallucinations for the past 6 weeks. During the past month he displayed pressured and disorganized speech. He was also grandiose, talked incessantly, was hyperactive and distractible, and went for long periods without sleep. He has been unable to accomplish his academic work and has been disruptive in class.

205. With this patient, it would be important to investigate the possibility of substance abuse, and the most likely substance would be

(A) alcohol
(B) stimulants, such as cocaine or amphetamine
(C) benzodiazepines, such as diazepam (Valium)
(D) narcotics
(E) tricyclic antidepressants

206. The most likely diagnosis would be

(A) schizophrenia
(B) schizoaffective disorder
(C) delusional disorder
(D) bipolar I disorder
(E) schizoid personality disorder

207. The patient's medical condition would require evaluation, in that any of the following medical illnesses can result in psychotic symptoms EXCEPT

(A) cerebral neoplasm
(B) hypothyroidism
(C) hyperthyroidism
(D) asthma
(E) hepatic or renal disease

208. Any of the following drugs might be used to treat the patient's psychotic symptoms EXCEPT

(A) benzodiazepines
(B) lithium
(C) chlorpromazine
(D) olanzapine
(E) haloperidol

209. True statements about risperidone include all the following EXCEPT

(A) it is used in the treatment of schizophrenia
(B) it is a D_2 antagonist
(C) it may be associated with insomnia
(D) it is usually prescribed in dosages of about 6 mg/day
(E) it is associated with a high incidence of tardive dyskinesia

210. Which of the following statements regarding thought disorder is true?

(A) It is invariably found in schizophrenia
(B) It is sometimes exhibited by patients with mania
(C) It is sometimes exhibited by patients with panic disorder
(D) It is reflected in the speech but not the written communication of schizophrenics
(E) It is a phenomenon of schizophrenia first described by Sigmund Freud

211. Which of the following statements regarding delusions is true?

(A) Delusions are almost exclusively found in schizophrenia
(B) Delusions of grandiosity are rarely encountered except in mania
(C) Delusions involve a disturbance of cognition
(D) Delusions involve a disturbance of perception
(E) Delusions are a type of hallucination

212. In the absence of other symptoms, sporadically occurring behavioral automatisms and olfactory hallucinations suggest a diagnosis of

(A) schizophrenia
(B) hysterical personality disorder
(C) schizophreniform psychosis
(D) nondominant parietal lobe lesion
(E) temporal lobe lesion

213. Positive schizophrenic symptoms include all the following EXCEPT

(A) hallucinations
(B) delusions
(C) flattening of affect
(D) marked incoherence
(E) bizarre or disorganized behavior

214. In the catatonic form of schizophrenia, the clinical picture is dominated by at least two of the following features EXCEPT

(A) waxy flexibility or stupor
(B) marked paranoid delusions
(C) excessive motor activity
(D) extreme negativism
(E) echolalia or echopraxia

Items 215–216

215. Clozapine (Clozaril) is a drug used to relieve chronic symptoms of

(A) bipolar disorder
(B) major depression
(C) chronic schizophrenia
(D) Alzheimer's disease
(E) panic disorder

216. The most common side effects associated with clozapine include all the following EXCEPT

(A) extrapyramidal effects
(B) sedation
(C) agranulocytosis
(D) hypersalivation
(E) seizures

217. Which of the following statements is true about the likelihood of relapse in the long-term treatment of schizophrenia with neuroleptic medication?

(A) Relapse is more likely with oral than injectable neuroleptics
(B) After 1 year the relapse rate is about one-third
(C) The relapse rate is higher in more intelligent patients
(D) Nearly all patients will relapse within 5 years
(E) None of the above

218. Which of the following drugs may induce a psychosis that is easily confused with, or misdiagnosed as, paranoid schizophrenia?

(A) Barbiturates
(B) Heroin
(C) Benzodiazepines
(D) Amphetamines
(E) Chlorpromazine

219. In a typical year, out of a cohort of 10,000, the number of persons 15 years of age or older who will develop a schizophrenic illness for the first time is

(A) 1
(B) 5
(C) 10
(D) 50
(E) 100

220. In the criteria set forth by DSM-IV which of the following would distinguish schizophrenia from a manic episode?

(A) The schizophrenic patient will exhibit evidence of a thought disorder
(B) The manic patient is persistently elated, whereas the schizophrenic patient displays blunted, flat, or inappropriate affect
(C) The schizophrenic's psychosis is most often treated with neuroleptic medication
(D) The schizophrenic's psychosis is episodic while mania is generally continuous
(E) None of the above

221. Correct statements regarding the diagnostic criteria for delusional (paranoid) disorder, according to DSM-IV, include all the following EXCEPT

(A) auditory or visual hallucinations, if present, are not prominent
(B) behavior is not bizarre
(C) delusions are bizarre
(D) any associated affective syndrome is of brief duration relative to the duration of the delusional disturbance
(E) an organic factor has not initiated and maintained the disturbance

222. It has been demonstrated that lower socioeconomic status is associated with a higher prevalence rate for schizophrenia. True statements concerning this relationship include all the following EXCEPT

(A) it has been attributed to the effects of downward social mobility secondary to the illness
(B) it has been attributed to social and health conditions within lower socioeconomic environments
(C) it is supported by prevalence rates two or more times higher than those found in higher socioeconomic groups
(D) it is supported by the finding that the prevalence rate is higher in immigrant populations
(E) it has been demonstrated within the United States, but not within Europe

223. The percentage of schizophrenic patients who ultimately commit suicide is approximately

(A) 1 percent
(B) 5 percent
(C) 10 percent
(D) 20 percent
(E) 30 percent

224. True statements about delusional disorder include all the following EXCEPT

(A) delusional disorder is highly related to schizophrenic disorder
(B) delusional disorder is unrelated to depressive disorder
(C) premorbidly the patients tend to be more extroverted
(D) the incidence is equal in homosexual and heterosexual persons
(E) the delusions are well systematized and nonbizarre

225. Studies of the relationship between gender and schizophrenia have generally demonstrated that

(A) the usual age of onset is earlier for females than males
(B) males tend to have a better prognosis than females
(C) the lifetime risk of developing schizophrenia is approximately the same in males and females
(D) males tend to respond better to neuroleptic medication
(E) there is a higher concordance rate in male monozygotic twins as compared with female monozygotic twins

226. The mental status examination of patients with schizophrenia most commonly demonstrates a marked disorder of

(A) orientation
(B) memory
(C) mood
(D) thinking
(E) insight

227. The diagnosis of schizoaffective disorder includes all the following EXCEPT

(A) the condition includes the characteristic symptoms of schizophrenia
(B) the condition includes major depressive symptoms or a manic episode
(C) the condition includes delusions or hallucinations in the absence of prominent mood symptoms
(D) symptoms of a mood episode are present during much of the illness
(E) the condition can occur in response to the effects of a substance

DIRECTIONS: Each group of questions below consists of lettered options followed by numbered items. For each numbered item, select the appropriate lettered option(s). Each lettered option may be used once, more than once, or not at all. **Choose exactly the number of options indicated following each item.**

Items 228–231

Match each concept with the correct name.

(A) Emil Kraepelin
(B) Eugen Bleuler
(C) Harry Stack Sullivan
(D) Frieda Fromm-Reichmann
(E) Sigmund Freud

228. The schizophrenogenic mother. **(SELECT 1 NAME)**

229. Dementia praecox renamed schizophrenia. **(SELECT 1 NAME)**

230. Interpersonal theory of schizophrenia. **(SELECT 1 NAME)**

231. The symptoms of schizophrenia (dementia praecox) delineated on the basis of course and outcome. **(SELECT 1 NAME)**

Items 232–235

For each experience related to body function, select the correct diagnosis.

(A) Koro
(B) Delusional disorder
(C) Body dysmorphic disorder
(D) Delirium tremens
(E) Schizophreniform disorder

232. The conviction that parasites are crawling within the skin, but general behavior not obviously odd or bizarre. **(SELECT 1 DIAGNOSIS)**

233. Belief that one's genitals are being retracted into the body. **(SELECT 1 DIAGNOSIS)**

234. Visions involving extraterrestrials using a weapon to shoot parasites into the body, which causes unbearable itching. **(SELECT 1 DIAGNOSIS)**

235. Frightening visual hallucinations of being attacked by bugs in a patient with a clouded sensorium. **(SELECT 1 DIAGNOSIS)**

Schizophrenia and Other Psychotic Disorders

Answers

205–208. The answers are 205-B, 206-B, 207-D, 208-A. *(Isselbacher, 13/e, pp 2414–2417.)* A wide variety of substances can produce psychotic symptoms with either abuse or overdose. The stimulant drugs, notably cocaine and amphetamine, are particularly apt to produce a psychotic disorder with paranoid symptomatology. This psychosis is often hard to distinguish from schizophrenia, though it is usually present for a shorter duration than that required for the diagnosis of schizophrenia.

The patient displays the symptoms of schizophrenia and meets the criterion of a disturbance of at least 6 months' duration with at least 1 month of symptoms, including at least two or more of the following: hallucinations, delusions, disorganized speech or behavior, or negative symptoms. In addition, however, the patient displayed prominent manic symptomatology, such as grandiosity and hyperactivity, during the month prior to hospitalization. The patient therefore meets the criteria for a diagnosis of schizoaffective disorder. Patients with schizoid personality disorder do not show psychotic symptomatology, and patients with delusional disorder do not display bizarre delusions. Bipolar manic disorder is often hard to differentiate from schizophrenia, but such patients generally do not have a history of periods of psychosis that are without prominent mood symptoms.

Many medical illnesses can be associated with psychotic disorders and may at times be confused with schizophrenia, schizoaffective disorder, or mood disorders. These include neoplasms, endocrine disorders, cardiovascular disease, and renal and hepatic disease, as well as a host of other conditions. Asthma is not associated with psychotic symptoms.

Chlorpromazine was one of the earliest antipsychotic medications, and olanzapine is one of the newest. Haloperidol is also commonly prescribed. Lithium is frequently used to treat mood disorders, particularly manic symptomatology. Benzodiazepines may be used to combat anxiety but are not considered antipsychotic medications.

209. The answer is E. *(Gabbard, p 978.)* Risperidone is an antipsychotic medication often used in the treatment of schizophrenia. It has a potency as a D_2 antagonist comparable to that of haloperidol. The majority of patients are maintained on a dosage approximating 6 mg/day, with insomnia, agitation and extrapyramidal symptoms being common adverse effects. It is not a drug associated with a high incidence of tardive dyskinesia.

210. The answer is B. *(Hales, 2/e, pp 418–419.)* The abnormalities found in schizophrenic speech and writing were originally best described by Kraepelin and Bleuler. While these were originally considered to be a hallmark of that illness, modern investigation and clinical experience have shown that they can also be exhibited by patients with other psychiatric disorders, such as mania. Thought disorder is commonly found in schizophrenia, but there are significant numbers of patients who do not demonstrate the phenomenon. A disturbance in thinking is but one of a number of features associated with this diagnosis.

211. The answer is C. *(Hales, 2/e, p 214.)* Delusions are found in a wide variety of psychotic conditions other than schizophrenia, including organic disorders and some mood disorders. A delusion is defined as a firmly held belief that is untrue and contrary to a person's educational and cultural background. The patient clings to the belief even in the face of great contrary evidence. The delusions of schizophrenia show a wide variety of themes, but no particular theme is specific to either schizophrenia or any other mental disorder. While grandiose delusions are a common finding in mania, they are also found in other conditions. Hallucinations are disorders of perception.

212. The answer is E. *(Yudofsky, 2/e, p 482.)* While there are numerous reports of schizophrenic-like illness in patients with temporal lobe tumors, in fact their psychotic symptoms are usually atypical for classic schizophrenia. Commonly these patients present with mood swings, suicidal ideation, and olfactory, visual, or tactile hallucinations in addition to the typical auditory hallucinations of schizophrenia. Most often one sees "spells" of difficulty, and an absence of the usual affect disturbance and interpersonal difficulties of schizophrenia. Not infrequently patients with temporal lobe tumors will present with depressed mood, mania, or hypomania.

213. The answer is C. *(Hales, 2/e, pp 420–421.)* Clinicians commonly find it useful to separate positive and negative symptoms in schizophrenia. All those mentioned are positive symptoms, except for flattening of affect. This is a negative symptom, along with other reflections of a deficiency of mental functioning such as poverty of speech, anhedonia, anergia, and the absence of social contacts.

214. The answer is B. *(Hales, 2/e, p 425.)* In catatonic schizophrenia the clinical picture must be dominated by at least two of the stated symptoms, with the exception of paranoid delusions. These are especially prominent in paranoid schizophrenia. Immobility may be expressed by catalepsy, waxy flexibility, or stupor, and excessive activity by seemingly purposeless, excessive motor behavior.

215–216. The answers are 215-C, 216-A. *(Schatzberg, pp 631–632.)* Clozapine (Clozaril) is one of the newer drugs that has shown much promise in the treatment of chronically and severely ill schizophrenic patients. This includes many patients who have been treatment-resistant with respect to standard antipsychotic medications. Improvement has been noted in both negative and positive symptoms. Careful monitoring is essential because a small but significant percentage of patients may develop potentially fatal agranulocytosis. Another potentially serious side effect is seizure. Other common problems include sedation, hypersalivation, tachycardia, constipation, and effects on blood pressure. The lower incidence of extrapyramidal side effects and the absence of tardive dyskinesia have been of great interest.

217. The answer is B. *(Hales, 2/e, pp 615–634.)* While reported results vary widely, over the past 2 decades most studies suggest that about one-third of schizophrenic patients will have a recurrence of their psychosis despite maintenance on neuroleptic medication. Such medication clearly reduces, but does not eliminate, the risk of relapse. Relapse rates have been similar even in studies in which compliance is controlled through the use of longitudinal injectable medication. There are significant numbers of patients who do not relapse when followed over many years. The decision for long-term drug maintenance therapy is a complex one that must weigh benefits versus the risk of serious side effects.

218. The answer is D. *(Hales, 2/e, p 394.)* Abuse of amphetamines can result in a psychosis very closely resembling acute paranoid schizophrenia. Symptoms include paranoid delusions and visual hallucinations. Some investigators feel that prominent visual hallucinations and a relative absence of thought disorder are more characteristic of amphetamine psychosis, but other investigators feel the symptoms are indistinguishable. Other drugs that produce psychoses similar to schizophrenia include phencyclidine (PCP) and lysergic acid diethylamide (LSD).

219. The answer is A. *(Hales, 2/e, pp 431–432.)* Determining the epidemiology of schizophrenia is a difficult process because of enormous differences in such factors as case finding and definitions. However, it appears that in a typical year about 1 person in 10,000 who are age 15 or older will develop a schizophrenic illness for the first time. The lifetime prevalence is about 100 per 10,000 for persons who survive into their late fifties.

220. The answer is E. *(DSM-IV, pp 274–286, 342–345. Hales, 2/e, pp 417–423.)* None of the distinctions set forth in this question apply to the disorders. An affective diagnosis may be associated with "first rank" symptoms such as thought broadcasting or thought insertion, and similarly, the presence of mood-incongruent delusions or hallucinations, in the absence of a full affective syndrome, may point toward schizophrenia. While it is true that in schizophrenia there must be continuous signs of illness for at least 6 months, this need not be continuous psychosis but may include prodromal or residual symptoms. Mania is usually episodic, but chronicity of psychosis does not exclude the diagnosis of mania if other criteria are fulfilled. It is true that most often mania is treated by lithium, but neuroleptic medication is commonly used with both schizophrenia and the acute phases of mania. Also, treatment methodology is not part of the diagnostic criteria.

221. The answer is C. *(DSM-IV, pp 296–301.)* The delusions in delusional disorder are not bizarre. This fact helps to differentiate the condition from paranoid schizophrenia or schizophreniform disorder, in which delusions are usually bizarre and hallucinations are often present. In delusional disorder, the delusions usually involve situations that occur in real life, such as being followed, poisoned, loved at a distance, and so on.

222. The answer is E. *(Hales, 2/e, p 433.)* Higher incidence and prevalence of schizophrenia have been found repeatedly to occur in association with lower socioeconomic conditions, whether urban or rural. The evidence is more striking in large urban centers. This has been demonstrated both in Europe and the United States. Depending on the study, the incidence has been reported to be as much as six times higher in lower socioeconomic groups. Some feel this relationship is causal—that it is due to such factors as social isolation, poor prenatal care, and the stress of poverty. There is probably better evidence for the hypothesis that the relationship is due to downward social drift as a consequence of the impaired motivation, social skills, cognition, and employability secondary to the illness.

223. The answer is C. *(Hales, 2/e, p 1256.)* Of all suicide victims, about 2 to 3 percent will have schizophrenia. It is estimated that about 10 percent of schizophrenic patients will ultimately commit suicide. The risk factors are generally believed to be male sex, age under 30, chronic illness and unemployment, a relapsing course, a high level of education, and depressive symptoms. Clinicians need to be particularly cognizant of the fact that schizophrenic patients who commit suicide often use very lethal means and fail to communicate their intent.

224. The answer is A. *(Hales, 2/e, p 453.)* Delusional disorder appears to be unrelated to either schizophrenia or to affective disorder. Prior to the onset of their illness these patients appear to be more extroverted, dominant, and hypersensitive than are schizophrenic patients, who tend to be schizoid or submissive. Freud believed that the persecutory delusions were related to unconscious homosexual conflict, while modern psychodynamic formulations are more apt to be related to issues of self-esteem. There is no increased incidence of delusional disorder in homosexual persons. Typically, the delusions of these patients are well systematized, nonbizarre, and related to situations that might occur in real life (e.g., being followed or poisoned).

225. The answer is C. *(Kaplan, 6/e, pp 432–433.)* Gender differences in schizophrenia have been repeatedly demonstrated. The lifetime risk for schizophrenia is the same in males and females, but males tend to have an earlier peak age of onset (18 to 25 years versus 26 to 45 years for females) and a poorer outcome. Females appear to be more responsive to neuroleptics, and in monozygotic twin studies, the concordance rates are higher in females than in males.

226. The answer is D. *(DSM-IV, pp 274–280.)* One common clinical finding during the mental status examination of a patient with schizophrenia is the presence of a thinking disorder. This may be a disorder of thought processes or content or both. Common findings include looseness of associations, autistic thinking, a failure of the ability to abstract, and delusional ideation. One certainly can encounter disturbances of mood and a lack of insight, but these are not hallmark features of the diagnosis. When cognition and memory disturbances seem to be present, they are usually secondary to the patient's agitation, autism, and thought disorder.

227. The answer is E. *(DSM-IV, pp 292–296.)* The diagnosis of schizoaffective disorder is one of the most confusing in psychiatric nosology. The criteria indicate that there must be an uninterrupted illness during which, at some time, there is either a major depressive or manic episode along with the characteristic symptoms of schizophrenia. Additionally, there must be delusions or hallucinations for at least 2 weeks that are not in response to the mood symptoms. When the above is in response to a substance, as in substance abuse, the diagnosis cannot be made.

228–231. The answers are 228-D, 229-B, 230-C, 231-A. *(Hales, 2/e, pp 412–414.)* Emil Kraepelin (1828-1899) carefully studied the course and outcome of seriously mentally ill patients. He noted that some had symptoms such as delusions and withdrawal at a relatively early age and were likely to have a chronic and deteriorating course. To distinguish these patients with "dementia" at an early age from those with late-onset dementias, Alzheimer's disease, and manic-depressive illness, he referred to the disorder as dementia praecox.

Bleuler (1857-1939) also observed patients over long periods of time and became convinced that a thought disorder that involved a "splitting" of cognitive functions was the pathognomonic feature of this disorder. He renamed the condition schizophrenia

Sigmund Freud felt that these patients were untreatable by psychoanalysis because of their severe libidinal regression, which made them unable to form relationships and, in particular, a transference.

Sullivan saw schizophrenia not so much in intrapsychic terms but as a result of environmental influence in which the patient had an insufficient developmental exposure to positive interpersonal relationships.

Fromm-Reichmann believed that schizophrenia was the outcome of an inadequate mother-child relationship in which the mother was aloof, overly protective, or hostile.

232–235. The answers are 232-B, 233-A, 234-E, 235-D. *(DSM-IV, pp 445–449. Kaplan, 6/e, p 1056.)* Koro is a condition reported mainly in China, Malaysia, and Thailand that involves intense anxiety that one's genitals are retracting into the body. Males may attach devices to the penis to prevent the retraction, and females are concerned with the vulva or breasts. The patient believes that if the genitals become fully retracted into the abdomen, he or she will die.

Delusions involving bugs are common to a number of psychiatric disorders. Bizarre bodily delusions, in the absence of an organic disorder, most commonly are associated with the diagnosis of schizophrenia or schizophreniform disorder. The latter has features identical to those of schizophrenia, but the duration is less than 6 months.

Prominent hallucinations are not present in delusional (paranoid) disorder, and the general behavior is not obviously odd or bizarre. Patients with the somatic type of delusional disorder usually consult nonpsychiatric physicians for treatment of their perceived somatic condition.

Alcohol withdrawal delirium (delirium tremens) by definition is associated with global cognitive impairment and is often associated with vivid hallucinations, delusions, and agitated behavior. Global cognitive impairment is not found in the other conditions discussed above.

Body dysmorphic disorder involves preoccupation, not delusion.

Mood Disorders

DIRECTIONS: Each item below contains a question or incomplete statement followed by suggested responses. Select the **one best** response to each question.

Items 236–237

A 55-year-old man is admitted to a general hospital for the treatment of cardiac symptoms. He has a history of myocardial infarction and ventricular arrhythmia and currently has been diagnosed with an early major depression.

236. All the following treatments would be reasonable considerations for a man with this cardiac history EXCEPT

(A) electroconvulsive therapy (ECT)
(B) bupropion
(C) fluoxetine
(D) sertraline
(E) imipramine

237. One would need to use care in prescribing a monoamine oxidase (MAO) inhibitor because of potential

(A) nausea
(B) major effects on cardiac conduction
(C) orthostatic hypotension
(D) induction of mania
(E) sexual side effects

238. Studies of bipolar illness show an average concordance rate in monozygotic twins of about

(A) 5 percent
(B) 20 percent
(C) 50 percent
(D) 80 percent
(E) 95 percent

239. The occurrence of depression, as an early symptom, has been particularly associated with carcinoma of the

(A) prostate
(B) bladder
(C) parathyroid
(D) pancreas
(E) ovary

240. In the treatment of an 85-year-old man with major depression, which of the following medications would be LEAST likely to be used?

(A) Fluoxetine
(B) Doxepin
(C) Sertraline
(D) Desipramine
(E) Nortriptyline

241. A 27-year-old woman seeks evaluation for her "depression" in an outpatient clinic. She reports episodic feelings of sadness since adolescence. Occasionally she feels good, but these periods seldom last more than 2 weeks. She is able to work but thinks she is not doing as well as she should. In describing her problems, she seems to focus more on repeated disappointments in her life and her low opinion of herself than on discrete depressive symptoms. In your differential diagnosis at this point, the most likely diagnosis is

(A) major depression with melancholia
(B) adjustment disorder with depressed mood
(C) cyclothymia
(D) childhood depression
(E) dysthymia

242. The antidepressant medication most commonly associated with priapism is

(A) trazodone
(B) doxepin
(C) sertraline
(D) clomipramine
(E) imipramine

Items 243–244

One month after her mother's death from chronic heart disease, a 25-year-old woman with no prior psychiatric history has the onset of irritability, difficulty concentrating, sudden fits of crying, and difficulty falling asleep.

243. The most likely diagnosis would be

(A) major depression
(B) dysthymia
(C) posttraumatic stress disorder
(D) adjustment disorder
(E) uncomplicated bereavement

244. Appropriate possible treatment approaches include all the following EXCEPT

(A) antidepressant medication
(B) neuroleptic medication
(C) short-term psychodynamic psychotherapy
(D) support groups
(E) cognitive psychotherapy

245. The cognitive functioning of a person with a major depression is often characterized by all the following manifestations EXCEPT

(A) bizarre associations
(B) suicidal ideation
(C) obsessive rumination
(D) concentration impairment
(E) memory impairment

246. All the following are sometimes used in treatment-resistant depression to augment failed antidepressant treatment EXCEPT

(A) lithium
(B) thyroid medication
(C) dopaminergic agents
(D) steroids
(E) stimulants

247. The prevalence of clinical depression among poststroke patients is

(A) 1 to 2 percent
(B) 10 to 15 percent
(C) 30 to 50 percent
(D) 75 to 80 percent
(E) 90 to 100 percent

248. The basis for the therapeutic effect of electroconvulsive therapy (ECT) is

(A) seizure activity
(B) electrical stimulation of the brain
(C) memory loss
(D) the depressed patient's wish for punishment
(E) the depressed patient's attitude toward ECT

249. Following a stroke, the high-risk period for depression extends for

(A) 2 weeks
(B) 1 to 2 months
(C) 6 months
(D) 1 year
(E) 2 years

250. "Maternity blues" is accurately characterized by which of the following?

(A) It is more acute than postpartum depression
(B) It is usually a chronic and relapsing syndrome
(C) It affects 50 to 80 percent of all new mothers
(D) It is characterized by persistent apathy
(E) It is not associated with sleep disturbance

251. All the following endocrine conditions are commonly associated with depression EXCEPT

(A) hypoprolactinemia
(B) hypothyroidism
(C) hyperthyroidism
(D) Cushing's syndrome
(E) hyperparathyroidism

252. The percentage of new mothers who develop postpartum depression is believed to be approximately

(A) 0.5 to 1 percent
(B) 10 to 15 percent
(C) 25 to 30 percent
(D) 35 to 40 percent
(E) in excess of 50 percent

253. Among seriously depressed patients, the proportion that can be expected eventually to commit suicide is

(A) less than 1 percent
(B) about 2 percent
(C) about 15 percent
(D) about 30 percent
(E) about 60 percent

254. All the following statements about suicide are true EXCEPT

(A) it is among the top 10 leading causes of death in the United States
(B) it is almost always associated with illness, especially depression
(C) it has a significant familial incidence
(D) it is more apt to be completed in males than in females
(E) it is less likely in persons who have communicated their intent to others

255. While delusions of any variety can occur in major depressive disorder with psychotic features, the most common delusions are

(A) mood-incongruent
(B) mood-congruent
(C) mood-unrelated
(D) mood-controlling
(E) none of the above

256. All the following statements about people addicted to cocaine who binge until their supply is exhausted and then experience withdrawal are true EXCEPT

(A) the resulting "crash" begins 2 to 3 days following abstinence
(B) the crash lasts for about 3 days
(C) the person commonly experiences depression
(D) anxiety and irritability are common
(E) symptoms can be alleviated by medication

257. A 55-year-old married professor without a previous psychiatric history is early in her menopause. In addition to experiencing "hot flashes" and some irritability, she complains of episodes of dizzy spells and memory lapses, which she had experienced on several occasions earlier in life. She denies depressive symptoms either now or in the past. In particular, she should be evaluated for possible

(A) schizophrenia
(B) major depression
(C) temporal lobe epilepsy
(D) dysthymia
(E) panic disorder

258. A diagnosis of bipolar disorder might be appropriate for patients who have all the following EXCEPT

(A) recurrent depressions and a history of mania
(B) recurrent depressions without a history of mania
(C) mania now and a history of a depressive episode
(D) mania now without a history of past affective disturbances
(E) a history of several manic episodes without depression

259. Cyclothymia is distinguished from major affective disorder primarily by

(A) family history
(B) an absence of chronicity
(C) age of onset
(D) severity and duration of symptoms
(E) preexisting personality pattern

260. True statements about depression that occurs concomitantly with a medical illness include all the following EXCEPT

(A) it may be the result of medication
(B) it is usually unresponsive to antidepressant medication
(C) it may not be related to the medical illness
(D) it may be the first symptom of the medical illness to appear
(E) it may have the same signs and symptoms as endogenous depression

261. Which of the following disorders is an absolute contraindication to the use of electroconvulsive therapy (ECT)?

(A) Aortic aneurysm
(B) Brain tumor
(C) Coronary artery disease
(D) Pregnancy
(E) None of the above

262. The concept that psychopathology, including depression, is the result of developmental deficits related to self-esteem and the development of a cohesive self is associated with the psychoanalyst

(A) Franz Alexander
(B) Carl Jung
(C) Harry Stack Sullivan
(D) Heinz Kohut
(E) Sigmund Freud

263. The term double depression is used to describe

(A) a particularly severe bout of major depression
(B) major depression superimposed on dysthymia
(C) recurrent episodes of major depression within a 2-month period
(D) medical illness with a superimposed episode of major depression
(E) major depression superimposed on "maternity blues"

264. True statements about seasonal affective disorder include all the following EXCEPT

(A) it is more common in women than in men
(B) it may be associated with mood elevation
(C) symptoms often include hypersomnia and weight gain
(D) it is commonly treated with light therapy
(E) depression characteristically begins in the fall or winter

265. True statements about disturbance of sleep associated with mood disorders include all the following EXCEPT

(A) patients often complain of early morning awakening
(B) depressed patients with bipolar illness often complain of excessive sleep
(C) sleep latency (time from sleep onset to REM sleep) is often reduced
(D) sleep deprivation may induce a temporary remission of depression
(E) manic patients generally require excessive amounts of sleep because of their hyperactivity

266. While the majority of women do not experience significant side effects when taking oral contraceptives, for those who do, the most commonly encountered psychological problem is

(A) anxiety
(B) depression
(C) night terrors
(D) short-term memory defects
(E) long-term memory defects

DIRECTIONS: The group of questions below consists of lettered options followed by numbered items. For each numbered item, select the appropriate lettered option(s). Each lettered option may be used once, more than once, or not at all. **Choose exactly the number of options indicated following each item.**

Items 267–270

Each statement below refers to an etiologic theory of depression. Select the name most closely associated with each statement.

(A) Kraepelin
(B) Lewinsohn
(C) Abraham
(D) Beck
(E) Seligman

267. In contrast to the usual mourner's grief over the lost person, the depressed person is concerned with loss and guilt resulting from unconscious hostility toward the lost person. **(SELECT 1 NAME)**

268. Depression results from specific cognitive distortions present in depression-prone people. **(SELECT 1 NAME)**

269. Depression relates to "learned helplessness." **(SELECT 1 NAME)**

270. The depressed person lacks social skills, and a decrease in pleasant events or an increase in unpleasant events leads to dysphoria and self-blame, which are then reinforced by the environment. **(SELECT 1 NAME)**

Mood Disorders

Answers

236–237. The answers are 236-E, 237-C. *(Practice Guidelines [see under American Psychiatric Association in Bibliography], pp 114–115.)* The presence of cardiac disease complicates the treatment of depression. While cardiac disease is not an absolute contraindication to ECT, the more common initial treatment would be with antidepressants. The tricyclic antidepressants must be used with great care because of their potential effects on cardiac function, while bupropion and specific serotonin reuptake inhibitors (SSRIs) appear to be safe in most instances.

Monoamine oxidase inhibitors must be used with caution because they have the potential to induce orthostatic hypotension. They also pose a risk of adversely interacting with other medications taken by such patients. For this reason they would not be a first-line treatment.

238. The answer is D. *(Yudofsky, 2/e, pp 210–211.)* The evidence for a genetic factor in bipolar affective disorders is reasonably sound. The concordance rate for bipolar illness in monozygotic twins averages 80 percent when various studies are combined. The concordance rate in dizygotic twins and siblings is 29 percent, which is significantly higher than that found in the general population.

239. The answer is D. *(Rundell, pp 312–313.)* Carcinoma of the pancreas has long been associated with the occurrence of emotional disorder, and the most commonly described symptoms are depression and an intense sense of dread. The incidence of depression that predates the discovery of the malignancy varies from 10 to 50 percent. The symptoms are often similar to those of a major depressive episode, with or without vegetative signs.

240. The answer is B. *(Practice Guidelines, p 118.)* In the treatment of elderly patients, one must consider the fact that they are particularly prone to orthostatic hypotension and to cholinergic blockade. The latter is much more likely with doxepin than with the other agents. This would be even more of a concern if other potentiating medications were being taken by the patient.

241. The answer is E. *(DSM-IV, pp 345–349.)* Dysthymia is a chronic depression that lasts at least 2 years; it usually begins in late adolescence or early adulthood. Sometimes patients describe being depressed for as long as they can remember. Symptoms fluctuate but are usually not severe. Such patients are commonly concerned with their perceived failures or interpersonal disappointments. The somatic symptoms characteristic of major depression or melancholia are less prominent in dysthymia.

242. The answer is A. *(Yudofsky, 2/e, pp 667–669.)* Most antidepressants have been associated with sexual dysfunction, commonly reduced libido or difficulty in reaching orgasm. Trazodone has been known to cause priapism, usually within 3 days to 18 months. This is a potentially serious side effect.

243–244. The answers are 243-E, 244-B. *(DSM-IV, pp 684–685.)* Following the death of a loved one, a full depressive syndrome may occur as a normal response to the loss. This usually begins several weeks later and may last for up to a year, though for most it is mostly gone after 4 to 6 months. It is distinguished from major depression by the absence of morbid preoccupation with worthlessness, lesser functional impairment, and the usual absence of marked psychomotor retardation or delusions. For the patient described, dysthymia is an inappropriate diagnosis because of the absence of previous depressive trends. The symptoms are not those that meet the criteria for posttraumatic stress disorder, and bereavement is specifically excluded from the official diagnosis of adjustment disorder. All the indicated treatments are commonly used with the exception of neuroleptics, which are reserved for use as antipsychotic agents.

245. The answer is A. *(Kaplan, 6/e, pp 1128–1129.)* People with typical unipolar depression ruminate about guilt, suicide, somatic fears, or other depressive themes. Concentration and recent-memory impairment, which at first may suggest an organic brain syndrome, improve with the lifting of depression. Concentration and memory difficulties that are secondary to the depression also may be difficult to distinguish from the side effects of anti-depressant medication; thus, these symptoms should be carefully assessed before initiation of pharmacotherapy. Although the content of depressive thinking may be delusional or gruesome, the associations or connections characterizing the thought process of depressed persons are usually conventional and seldom bizarre.

246. The answer is D. *(Gabbard, 2/e, pp 1283–1289.)* In treatment-resistant depressions, common treatment strategies include augmenting treatment, using a higher dose of antidepressant, combining two classes of antidepressants, or switching to another antidepressant. Of the drugs mentioned, lithium is probably the most common means of augmentation, but thyroid medication, dopamine agonists (e.g., bromocriptine, pergolide), and stimulants have all been used with some success. Steroids are not used to augment treatment.

247. The answer is C. *(Rundell, pp 322–323.)* Estimates of the prevalence of clinical depression in poststroke patients range from 30 to 50 percent. This is not merely due to the effects of physical impairment, but also to intrinsic biological contributions such as injury to catecholamine pathways. There is a higher incidence of depression among patients with left rather than right hemispheric lesions, and especially left anterior lesions.

248. The answer is A. *(Kaplan, 6/e, pp 2130–2131.)* The therapeutic effect of ECT depends on the production of a seizure. (In fact, convulsions have a beneficial effect on depression, whether they are induced electrically or with medication.) Subconvulsive electrical stimuli can produce loss of consciousness and memory and may even meet a person's wish for punishment, but these results have no effect on the lifting of depression.

249. The answer is E. *(Rundell, pp 322–323.)* Studies of the course and prognosis of poststroke depression indicate that the high-risk period extends for 2 years. The presence of depression is associated with both higher morbidity and mortality. This underscores the importance of psychiatric intervention in poststroke patients.

250. The answer is C. *(Kaplan, 6/e, pp 1063–1064.)* "Maternity blues" is a transient condition that usually resolves after 2 to 3 weeks. It affects 50 to 80 percent of all new mothers within the first week following delivery and is distinct from postpartum depression. The latter is distinguished by its more severe symptoms and by the fact that it persists following the first postpartum month. Generally, maternity blues is characterized by emotional lability, tearfulness, irritability, sleep disturbance, fatigue, and sometimes mild confusion.

251. The answer is A. *(Rundell, pp 327–329.)* Endocrine disorders are commonly associated with depression. Hyperprolactinemia, rather than hypoprolactinemia, is associated with both seizure disorder and depression and is usually due to hormone-secreting tumor, neuroleptic medication, pregnancy, oral contraceptives, renal failure, hypothyroidism, or cirrhosis. Major depressive episodes are seen in as many as 30 percent of patients with hyperthyroidism or hyperparathyroidism, and not infrequently in patients with hypothyroidism. Exogenous steroids may be associated with manic syndromes, but as many as two-thirds of patients with Cushing's syndrome have been reported to have clinical depression.

252. The answer is B. *(Kaplan, 6/e, p 1063.)* Postpartum depression is a much more common condition than is generally realized. It occurs in about 10 to 15 percent of new mothers. While it may initially resemble "maternity blues," it is distinguished by its persistence and severity. When psychotic symptoms are present, hospitalization may be required, and one must evaluate the possible need to protect the newborn child.

253. The answer is C. *(Practice Guidelines, p 107.)* Suicide is an ever-present danger in seriously depressed persons. The clinician must constantly be on the alert for the signs and symptoms of potential suicide, even in patients who appear to be responding to treatment. It is estimated that approximately 15 percent of seriously depressed persons will eventually kill themselves.

254. The answer is E. *(Hales, 2/e, pp 1251–1254, 1264–1265.)* Suicide is the ninth leading cause of death in the United States and is most often preventable. The vast majority of victims suffer from psychiatric illness, and the most common is mood disorder. Mood disorder has been identified in 40 to 80 percent of a consecutive series of suicides, and alcoholism in 20 to 30 percent. Males tend to be more successful than females in their attempts, and there is a clear familial association. It is estimated that up to 80 percent of suicide victims have communicated their intent to others, and thus such communications must be taken very seriously.

255. The answer is B. *(DSM-IV, pp 320–327.)* When delusions or hallucinations are present in major depressive disorder, the delusional content is usually congruent with the patient's mood. Since patients with major depression are often filled with guilt and feelings of worthlessness, it is not surprising that their delusions most commonly involve persecution because of some moral transgression or inadequacy. Other mood-congruent delusions encountered are nihilistic or somatic delusions and delusions of poverty. Symptoms due to mood-incongruent delusions are not included in the diagnostic criteria for a major depressive episode.

256. The answer is A. *(Rundell, p 332.)* The "crash" associated with cocaine withdrawal usually begins within hours of abstinence. It generally is characterized by depression, irritability, and anxiety, and it typically lasts about 3 days. The depressive symptoms are believed caused by central nervous system dopamine and norepinephrine depletion. Several drugs have been shown to attenuate the depressive symptoms, including bromocriptine, amantadine, and desipramine.

257. The answer is C. *(Yudofsky, 2/e, p 401.)* In contrast to popular opinion, there is no increase in the rate of depression or somatic symptoms during the menopause. However, complaints of hot flashes, fatigue, irritability, or depressive feelings are by no means uncommon. A complaint of memory lapses is not common in either panic or depressive disorders, and the absence of typical symptoms or history makes major depression or schizophrenia unlikely. This woman should have an EEG examination to rule out possible temporal lobe epilepsy. Her symptoms are consistent with psychomotor epilepsy, a condition that can be exacerbated at menopause.

258. The answer is B. *(DSM-IV, p 350.)* The bipolar-unipolar distinction is made entirely on the basis of mania. A current manic episode or a history of manic or hypomanic symptoms is necessary for the diagnosis of a bipolar disorder. The bipolar category is classified as depressed, manic, or mixed depending on the clinical presentation. The term unipolar is not part of official classification but is used by some clinicians for recurrent major depression.

259. The answer is D. *(DSM-IV, pp 363–365.)* Cyclothymia is a relatively common condition whose symptoms, family history, and response to treatment strongly suggest that it is a variant of bipolar disorder. The clinical course is chronic, and after two years, many patients have a major affective disorder. Except for the severity and duration of the irregularly alternating depressive and hypomanic periods, the clinical picture is quite similar to that seen in bipolar disorder.

260. The answer is B. *(Rundell, pp 312–318.)* While it is true that depression may be the first manifestation of a medical illness, it is equally true that the discovery of a medical illness does not necessarily explain the genesis of the depression. On a symptom basis, depression secondary to medical illness is often indistinguishable from primary depression. The treatment of medical illness may be a primary cause of depression, as, for example, depression secondary to steroid medication. Depression may also occur secondary to the consequences of the illness, for example, loss of autonomy and self-esteem or negative effects on personal and vocational life. When there are symptoms of a major depression, most patients will have a favorable response to the use of antidepressants.

261. The answer is E. *(Gabbard, 2/e, p 1246.)* There is no absolute contraindication to the use of ECT, but there are a number of conditions in which important risk factors must be weighed against the danger of untreated depression or depression unresponsive to treatment. The literature sometimes describes brain tumor to be an absolute contraindication because of the risk of brainstem herniation from increased intracranial pressure. However, there is growing evidence that with proper technique and medical management, these patients can safely undergo ECT. Bradycardia, tachycardia, hypertension, and increased cardiac work may occur during a seizure, and this may require modification in anesthetic technique to minimize the risk to patients with aneurysm or heart disease. A small series of case reports of ECT during pregnancy suggests that the procedure can be carried out with safety for both the mother and the fetus.

262. The answer is D. *(Kaplan, 6/e, pp 460–462.)* Heinz Kohut, originally a classical analyst, ultimately developed a theory of psychopathology that emphasized developmental deficit, as opposed to fixation and regression related to conflict regarding sexual and aggressive drives. He believed that the most important line of development related to the self, especially to self-esteem and self-cohesion. The development of a cohesive self requires phase-appropriate empathy in the form of mirroring and idealization from important objects ("self-objects"). Self-esteem is an important issue in many depressions.

263. The answer is B. *(Practice Guidelines, p 113.)* Patients with dysthymia may develop a major depression. When they do, this is sometimes referred to as double depression. Such patients are at greater risk for having a recurrence of a major depressive episode than are those patients who have major depression only.

264. The answer is B. *(Gabbard, 2/e, pp 1264–1267.)* Seasonal affective disorder has been recognized for quite some time, but the syndrome has been systematically investigated only in recent years. Patients are predominantly women, often with the depression and hypomania that has been associated with bipolar II disorder. The characteristic pattern is depression beginning in the fall and ending in the spring, often followed by euthymia, hypomania, or mania in the spring or summer. The depressive symptoms are often similar to those described by patients with atypical depression or bipolar illness, such as hypersomnia, carbohydrate craving, lack of energy, and weight gain. The common symptoms of depression—including hopelessness, depressed mood, and functional impairment—also occur.

265. The answer is E. *(Hales, 2/e, pp 846–847.)* There is an important relationship between depression and sleep disturbance. In major depression, sleep studies have shown a number of changes, including a shortened sleep latency and a shift of REM sleep such that more occurs in the earlier part of the night. Depressed patients almost always have sleep complaints, and these include difficulty in falling asleep, intermittent awakening, and early morning awakening. Patients with atypical depression or bipolar disorder typically display hypersomnia, but their sleep is not described as restful. During mania patients do not seem to require a normal amount of sleep and may describe going for long periods without sleep. Sleep deprivation has been shown to be capable of inducing a temporary remission in both major depression and bipolar disorder.

266. The answer is B. *(Hales, 2/e, p 1712.)* A great many studies have been done to determine the side effects of oral contraceptives, and the results are somewhat inconsistent. Most, however, suggest that the majority of women have no significant side effects. Many, but not all, studies report an increased incidence of depression.

267–270. The answers are 267-C, 268-D, 269-E, 270-B. *(Kaplan, 6/e, pp 1074, 1116–1117, 1182–1184.)* Kraepelin was a pioneer in the classification of psychiatric disorders early in this century. He emphasized the longitudinal history and pattern of symptoms. He differentiated what he called manic-depressive illness (major depression, bipolar disorder, and some patients with dysthymia) from dementia praecox (schizophrenia). He noted that the former had an episodic and relatively benign course, while the latter was often chronic and deteriorating.

Abraham (1911) was an early psychoanalytic theorist, who noted that unlike the usual mourner who grieves, the depressed person is preoccupied with guilt, loss, and inadequacy that are based on unconscious hostility toward the lost person. Freud (1917) expanded on these theories to note that, unlike the usual mourner, the depressed person is unable to resolve these ambivalent feelings. The anger toward the lost person is turned inward and results in dysphoria, guilt, and loss of self-esteem.

Lewinsohn (1974) proposed that the person who is likely to become depressed is one who lacks social skills. A subsequent decrease in response-contingent positive reinforcement (a decrease in pleasant events or an increase in unpleasant events) then leads to dysphoria and self-blame. Once the depression begins, the secondary gain (positive reinforcement from sympathy, attention, and so on) escalates the condition to the level of clinical depression.

Aaron Beck (1972) proposed a cognitive-behavioral model of depression. Depression-prone people have specific cognitive distortions ("depressogenic schemata") derived from early experience. These disturbed cognitions result in unrealistically negative views of self, world, and future.

Seligman proposed that experiences with uncontrollable events lead to cognitive and emotional deficits that result in a state of "learned-helplessness." The resultant expectations and conclusions about self and life events can result in depression.

Anxiety, Somatoform, and Dissociative Disorders

DIRECTIONS: Each item below contains a question or incomplete statement followed by suggested responses. Select the **one best** response to each question.

Items 271–272

A 42-year-old man is admitted to the hospital from the emergency room, brought in by a passerby who found him wandering, complaining of intense abdominal pain, strange sensations in his hands, and "amnesia." Physical examination reveals seven scars from previous abdominal surgery. He seems to relish the sick role and attention from the nurses, one of whom recognized him as someone who had appeared in several other hospital emergency rooms with complaints of abdominal pain. It was discovered that he was lying about his amnesia. He is demanding multiple diagnostic tests, including a liver biopsy. The mental status examination is unremarkable.

271. The most likely diagnosis is

(A) acute intermittent porphyria
(B) Munchausen syndrome
(C) malingering
(D) schizophrenia
(E) psychotic depression

272. This type of disorder is classified as

(A) somatoform
(B) dissociative
(C) adjustment
(D) factitious
(E) hysterical personality

273. Which of the following statements most correctly describes panic disorder?

(A) When associated with agoraphobia, it occurs more often in males than females
(B) No increased familial incidence has been identified
(C) The usual age of onset is in young adulthood
(D) It is often relieved by anxiolytic medications but not by antidepressants
(E) It often requires hospitalization for the initial phase of treatment

274. Depression and anxiety, with or without panic attacks, is seen in about half of patients with

(A) Cushing's syndrome
(B) hyponatremia
(C) hypernatremia
(D) hyperglycemia
(E) hypothyroidism

275. True descriptions of sleep panic include that it

(A) usually occurs during dreams
(B) is associated with REM activity
(C) occurs in many patients with panic disorder
(D) is associated with frightening difficulty in awakening
(E) has symptoms quite different from those of panic disorder

276. All the following statements about agoraphobia are true EXCEPT

(A) it is more common in females
(B) it is rarely accompanied by panic disorder
(C) it may result in the patient's being totally housebound
(D) it is frequently associated with a fear of being alone
(E) it often has an onset between 20 and 30 years of age

Items 277–279

A 23-year-old woman was seen in the emergency room stating that "out-of-the-blue" she was seized by intense fear associated with shortness of breath, a pounding heart, shaking, dizziness, a choking sensation, fear that she was dying or going crazy, and a desire to run away. The attack lasted about 20 min. This was the third occurrence of these symptoms in the past 3 weeks.

277. The most likely diagnosis is

(A) acute psychotic episode
(B) hypochondriasis
(C) panic attack
(D) generalized anxiety disorder
(E) major depression

278. Medical conditions commonly known to be associated with such symptomatology include all the following EXCEPT

(A) pheochromocytoma
(B) hypothyroidism
(C) hyperthyroidism
(D) hypoparathyroidism
(E) hyperparathyroidism
(F) hypoglycemia

279. All the following drugs are commonly employed in the pharmacological management of this patient's condition EXCEPT

(A) imipramine
(B) phenobarbital
(C) fluoxetine
(D) phenelzine
(E) alprazolam

280. All the following are true statements about multiple personality disorder EXCEPT

(A) the onset is usually in childhood
(B) there is often a history of childhood abuse
(C) the disorder is more common in females
(D) only one personality recurrently takes full control of the person's behavior
(E) the transition from one personality to another is often sudden

281. All the following statements about generalized anxiety disorder are true EXCEPT

(A) there is persistent anxiety lasting for at least 1 month
(B) the disorder is equally common in females and males
(C) the onset is usually in young adulthood
(D) symptoms include vigilance and scanning
(E) there is impairment of functioning

282. True statements about conversion disorder include all the following EXCEPT

(A) it may occur anytime from childhood to old age
(B) it is found more often in females
(C) prevalence rates in a general medical setting may reach 20 to 25 percent
(D) it occurs most frequently in upper socioeconomic groups
(E) it responds to a wide variety of treatment interventions

283. True statements about obsessive-compulsive disorder include all the following EXCEPT

(A) the onset is usually in adolescence or early adulthood
(B) patients attempt to neutralize thoughts or impulses by other thoughts or action
(C) anxiety is accentuated when a compulsion is carried out
(D) the disorder is found equally in men and women
(E) patients usually experience their compulsions or obsessions as intrusive and irrational

284. Obsessive-compulsive disorder

(A) usually has an onset in middle age
(B) has a lifetime prevalence of 0.1 percent
(C) is associated with greater concordance in monozygotic versus dizygotic twins
(D) is not responsive to pharmacological intervention
(E) has frequent spontaneous periods of complete remission

285. True statements about hyperventilation syndrome include all the following EXCEPT

(A) it may lead to respiratory acidosis
(B) it may produce a drop in serum calcium
(C) it is often associated with panic disorder
(D) it is associated with peripheral vasoconstriction
(E) it can be symptomatically reproduced by an infusion of sodium lactate

286. True statements about somatization disorder include all the following EXCEPT

(A) it has been called Briquet's syndrome
(B) it occurs more often in males
(C) it generally involves multiple somatic complaints
(D) it is most commonly seen in lower socioeconomic groups
(E) a familial pattern has been observed

287. Which of the following statements is true about the antianxiety drug buspirone (BuSpar)?

(A) It is a benzodiazepine
(B) It is particularly useful for the rapid treatment of acute anxiety states
(C) It is the most sedating of the commonly used antianxiety drugs
(D) On a per-milligram basis it is three times more potent than diazepam
(E) It has less potential for abuse than diazepam

288. All the following statements about pheochromocytoma tumors are true EXCEPT

(A) they may cause panic similar to spontaneous panic attacks
(B) they secrete catecholamines
(C) patients with pheochromocytoma rarely develop agoraphobia
(D) they are associated with malignant hypertensive episodes
(E) during an acute episode, patients generally demonstrate increased motor activity secondary to anxiety

289. Which of the following statements is true about postconcussional amnesia in contrast to dissociative (hysterical) amnesia?

(A) Postconcussional amnesia does not occur in combination with hysterical amnesia
(B) The retrograde amnesia following concussion generally does not extend beyond 1 week
(C) When postconcussional amnesia disappears, it does so rapidly and completely
(D) Hypnosis will commonly restore the lost memories of postconcussional amnesia
(E) It is usually factitious

290. According to DSM-IV, the diagnosis of hypochondriasis requires that the disorder have a duration of at least

(A) 1 month
(B) 3 months
(C) 6 months
(D) 1 year
(E) 3 years

291. All the following are true statements about depersonalization disorder EXCEPT

(A) reality testing remains intact during the depersonalization experience
(B) patients express the sense of being detached from their mental processes or body, or of being in a dreamlike state
(C) in the majority of patients it has a very slow and insidious onset
(D) it must be distinguished from occasional depersonalization, which is common and not necessarily pathological
(E) it must be distinguished from depersonalization secondary to brain tumor or temporal lobe epilepsy

DIRECTIONS: Each group of questions below consists of lettered options followed by numbered items. For each numbered item, select the appropriate lettered option(s). Each lettered option may be used once, more than once, or not at all. **Choose exactly the number of options indicated following each item.**

Items 292–294

Match each description to the appropriate phobia.

(A) Agoraphobia
(B) Social phobia
(C) Specific phobia
(D) None of the above

292. Generally elicited by a circumscribed stimulus.
(SELECT 2 PHOBIAS)

293. Characterized by marked fear and avoidance of being in places where help might not be available or escape not possible.
(SELECT 1 PHOBIA)

294. Characterized by persistent, irrational fear of humiliation or embarrassment.
(SELECT 1 PHOBIA)

Items 295–299

For each person, match the disorder.

(A) Somatization disorder
(B) Obsessive-compulsive disorder
(C) Dissociative fugue
(D) Body dysmorphic disorder
(E) Posttraumatic stress disorder

295. After watching her house burn down, a 32-year-old woman has recurrent dreams about the event.
(SELECT 1 DISORDER)

296. A 20-year old student is very upset because his nose looks crooked, though to others it appears normal. **(SELECT 1 DISORDER)**

297. A nun is found in a distant city working in a cabaret and is unable to remember her previous life. **(SELECT 1 DISORDER)**

298. A 35-year-old mother is anxious and upset by her inability to stop persistent impulses to stab her baby. **(SELECT 1 DISORDER)**

299. A college student has a 3-year history of episodes of amnesia and blindness, as well as multiple chest and gastrointestinal symptoms for which no organic cause can be found. **(SELECT 1 DISORDER)**

Anxiety, Somatoform, and Dissociative Disorders

Answers

271–272. The answers are 271-B, 272-D. *(Hales, 2/e, pp 623–632.)* Munchausen syndrome is an example of a very severe factitious disorder characterized by pathological lying, recurrent feigned or simulated illness, and wandering. Patients often display multiple scars from previous medical intervention and surgical exploration, and they will gladly submit to diagnostic procedures and operations. Acute intermittent porphyria is associated with abdominal pain, and sometimes psychiatric symptoms, but not those displayed by this patient. The absence of significant mental status findings, and particularly those associated with psychosis, eliminates schizophrenia and psychotic depression.

Factitious disorder is characterized by the feigning of physical or psychological symptoms and the motivation to assume the sick role. Patients with dissociative disorder, somatoform disorder, adjustment disorder, or hysterical personality may derive some secondary gain from their problems, but do not feign their illness. Malingering is the most difficult differential diagnosis. Malingering is distinguished from factitious disorders by the presence of an external incentive such as economic gain or avoidance of legal responsibility.

273. The answer is C. *(DSM-IV, pp 397–403.)* Panic disorder has an average age of onset in the twenties. Most studies suggest a higher rate in females. There is a clear familial trend, but there is controversy as to whether this is predominantly due to genetic or environmental influence. Both anxiolytic agents and antidepressants are often successful in the treatment of patients with this disorder. Effective treatment rarely requires initial hospitalization.

274. The answer is A. *(Yudofsky, 2/e, pp 519–538.)* The hypercortisolism of Cushing's syndrome is associated with depression and anxiety, with or without panic attacks, in about half of the patients. The picture often resembles that of a mixed manic and depressed state with considerable mood lability. Hyponatremia and hypernatremia result in prominent physical symptoms, and the neuropsychiatric manifestations usually relate to impaired cognition and ultimately impaired consciousness. Anxiety is not a predominant symptom in hypothyroidism, which usually involves depression and impaired cognition that sometimes leads to dementia or psychosis. Hyperglycemia presents mostly with physical symptoms such as polyuria, polydipsia, and polyphagia.

275. The answer is C. *(Kaplan, 6/e, p 848.)* As many as 70 percent of patients with panic disorder will report episodes of sleep panic. The typical history is of sudden awakening with symptoms similar to those of panic attacks that occur during the daytime. Reduced REM latency is not seen in panic disorder, and typically sleep panic occurs during non-REM sleep. It is not associated with either REM sleep or with dreaming.

276. The answer is B. *(DSM-IV, pp 397–405.)* Panic disorder with agoraphobia is more common than panic disorder without agoraphobia. However, occasionally patients will present with agoraphobia without a history or presence of panic disorder. In this condition the patient experiences the same fears of being in situations from which escape would be difficult, or in which help might not be available in the event that symptoms should develop. Commonly feared symptoms include becoming dizzy, loss of bladder or bowel control, and vomiting.

277–279. The answers are 277-C, 278-D, 279-B. *(Hales, 2/e, pp 495–518. Isselbacher, 13/e, pp 2165–2166.)* The patient displays typical symptoms of a panic attack: sudden onset of intense fear, with at least 4 of a potential 13 somatic or cognitive symptoms, and a duration of usually 5 to 20 min. Panic attacks can occur in a wide variety of psychiatric and medical conditions. The patient is diagnosed with panic disorder only if there are recurrent episodes of panic; there is at least 1 month of persistent concern, worry, or behavioral change associated with the attacks; and they are not due to the direct effect of medical illness or medication or substance abuse, or better accounted for by another psychiatric disorder. While anxiety can be intense in generalized anxiety disorder, major depression, acute psychosis, and hypochondriasis, it does not have the typical form described above. Phobias may be accompanied by situationally precipitated panic attacks.

A number of medical conditions can be accompanied by episodes of panic anxiety. These include pheochromocytoma, both hyper- and hypothyroidism, cardiac arrhythmias and coronary insufficiency, hypoglycemia, and both drug and alcohol withdrawal. Hypoparathyroidism is not associated with panic attacks, though there can be severe mental symptoms, including irritability, depression, and psychosis.

A number of pharmacologic agents have been used successfully in the treatment of patients with panic episodes or panic disorder. These include the tricyclic antidepressants (e.g., imipramine), serotonin reuptake inhibitors (e.g., fluoxetine, sertraline), monoamine oxidase inhibitors (e.g., phenelzine), and high-potency benzodiazepines (e.g., alprazolam, clonazepam). Phenobarbital is not an effective treatment for this condition and is further contraindicated because of concern about its addictive potential and sedative effects.

280. The answer is D. *(DSM-IV, pp 484–487.)* In adults, the number of personalities in any one case of multiple personality disorder varies from 2 to over 100. Approximately half of recently reported cases have 10 personalities or less. At least two of the personalities, at some time and recurrently, take full control of the person's behavior. The disorder often has its onset in childhood or adolescence, though commonly it is not diagnosed until later in life. Studies of patients with this disorder consistently reveal a high percentage who report having been subjected to sexual or physical abuse in childhood. In DSM-IV this condition is called dissociative identity disorder.

281. The answer is A. *(DSM-IV, pp 432–436.)* According to the criteria of DSM-IV, for a diagnosis of generalized anxiety disorder there must be symptoms of unrealistic or excessive anxiety about a number of life events or activities for 6 months or longer. The spectrum of symptoms includes signs of motor and muscle tension, fatigue, difficulty in concentration, irritability and sleep disturbance. The onset may be in childhood, adolescence, or young adulthood, the course is often chronic, and the disorder occurs a bit more often in females.

282. The answer is D. *(Hales, 2/e, pp 605–611.)* Conversion symptoms are very common in medical practice, and a prevalence rate of 20 to 25 percent has been estimated for patients admitted to a general medical setting. Conversion disorder is more common in females and can occur at any age. It is more frequent in less sophisticated, less educated patients with lower socioeconomic and rural backgrounds. Especially with early intervention, conversion symptoms tend to be short-lived and generally respond to a wide variety of interventions that involve suggestion of cure.

283. The answer is C. *(Hales, 2/e, pp 532–540.)* Typically patients with obsessive-compulsive disorder experience their symptoms as irrational, intrusive, and irresistible. They are aware that the problem is coming from their own mind and can usually acknowledge that the belief behind their action is unfounded or unreasonable. This is in contrast to the unshakable beliefs associated with delusions. When patients with this disorder attempt to stop compulsive behavior, tension and anxiety mount to the point where it is impossible to do so. Anxiety is therefore relieved by performing a compulsion.

284. The answer is C. *(Hales, 2/e, pp 532–544.)* Obsessive-compulsive disorder usually has its onset from late childhood to early adulthood and has a lifetime prevalence of about 2.5 percent. There is greater concordance in monozygotic versus dizygotic twins, suggesting a genetic contribution. While there are a minority of patients who have periods of complete remission, about one-third have a fluctuating course and up to 60 percent have a constant or progressive course. Many patients are markedly improved with pharmacological intervention. The most commonly used agents are serotonin reuptake inhibitors such as clomipramine, fluoxetine, and sertraline.

285. The answer is A. *(Kaplan, 6/e, pp 1501–1503.)* Episodes of hyperventilation are associated with rapid, shallow breathing; fear or panic; and frightening physical sensations. The hyperventilation induces a respiratory alkalosis through a loss of carbon dioxide. The attempt by the body to buffer this and maintain pH produces a drop in serum calcium (which can induce tetany) and also reflex vasoconstriction that affects the skin and central nervous system. Hyperventilation syndrome is often associated with the anxiety disorders, especially panic disorder. One can usually reproduce the patient's symptoms by experimental hyperventilation or by administering an infusion of sodium lactate.

286. The answer is B. *(Hales, 2/e, pp 594–602.)* Somatization disorder was formerly called hysteria and Briquet's syndrome. It consists of multiple somatic complaints, affects mostly women, and generally first appears in early adulthood. There is a familial pattern, and the disorder is more common among patients from lower socioeconomic backgrounds. It often coexists with other psychiatric disorders.

287. The answer is E. *(Gabbard, 2/e, p 2047.)* Buspirone has a chemical structure different from that of benzodiazepines and has a potency on a per-milligram basis that is equivalent to that of diazepam. It takes 1 to 2 weeks for the antianxiety effects to appear, so that it is not useful for anxiety conditions that require acute intervention. Buspirone is less sedating than the benzodiazepines and appears to have less potential for abuse.

288. The answer is E. *(Kaplan, 6/e, pp 1517–1518.)* Pheochromocytoma is a vascular tumor that produces catecholamines. Patients with this tumor can experience panic similar to that seen in patients with panic disorder. The diagnosis is suggested when there is a hypertensive response to smoking or malignant hypertensive episodes, crushing abdominal or back pain, or profuse sweating in the chest and back regions. Patients with anxiety disorders, including panic disorder, usually are hyperactive when anxious. Patients with pheochromocytoma characteristically want to stay very still during an episode of catecholamine release. The diagnosis can be confirmed by 24-h urine studies.

289. The answer is B. *(Kaplan, 6/e, pp 208–209, 1281–1285.)* Dissociative (hysterical) amnesia may occur following head injury, either alone or in combination with postconcussional amnesia. Typically the retrograde amnesia following concussion does not extend beyond 1 week, and the recovery of memories occurs slowly and in a spotty fashion. In contrast, the recovery from hysterical amnesia is usually sudden, dramatic, and complete. Hypnosis may be helpful as a diagnostic tool. If memories are restored during a hypnotic trance, it is likely that dissociative mechanisms are at least partially responsible for the amnesia.

290. The answer is C. *(Kaplan, 6/e, pp 462–465.)* Hypochondriasis is defined by DSM-IV as a condition in which there is a persistent fear or belief, despite medical reassurance, that one has a physical illness based upon misinterpretation of bodily symptoms. The belief is not of delusional proportions, and the patient's symptoms are not those of panic attacks. By definition the condition must persist for 6 months for this diagnosis to be made. It is estimated that from 3 to 14 percent of patients seen in a general medical practice may suffer from hypochondriasis.

291. The answer is C. *(Hales, 2/e, pp 641–642.)* The phenomenon of an occasional isolated depersonalization experience is quite common and occurs in both adults and children. To meet the diagnostic criteria for depersonalization disorder, as defined by DSM-IV, the experiences must be persistent and severe enough to cause distress, and reality testing must remain intact. In the majority of patients, symptoms appear suddenly, usually between the ages of 15 and 30. Since depersonalization can occur as a result of disturbed brain function, careful evaluation is necessary to rule out such diagnoses as brain tumor or temporal lobe epilepsy.

292–294. The answers are 292-B,C; 293-A; 294-B. *(DSM-IV, pp 403–417.)* Phobic disorders include agoraphobia, specific phobia, and social phobia. They are all characterized by overwhelming, persistent, and irrational fears that result in the overpowering need to avoid the object or situation that is generating the dread. Agoraphobia is the marked fear and avoidance of being alone or in public places where rapid exit would be difficult. As the phobia progresses, avoidance of the stimulus dominates the person's life. Social phobia is characterized by avoidance of situations in which one is exposed to scrutiny by others and a fear of being humiliated or embarrassed by one's actions. Specific phobias are triggered by objects (often animals), heights, or closed spaces. A large variety of objects are associated with simple phobias. Both social and specific phobias generally involve a circumscribed stimulus that elicits the phobic response.

295–299. The answers are 295-E, 296-D, 297-C, 298-B, 299-A. *(DSM-IV, pp 417–429, 446–450, 466–469, 481–484.)* One of the most characteristic features of posttraumatic stress disorder is the occurrence of repeated dreams or recollections of the traumatic event. There are numerous other symptoms, and the disturbance must persist for at least 1 month for the diagnosis to be made.

In body dysmorphic disorder, a person of normal appearance is preoccupied with some imaginary defect in appearance. The belief is tenacious, and sometimes of delusional intensity. The diagnosis specifically excludes anorexia nervosa (wherein patients who are thin often see themselves as fat) and transsexualism.

Patients with obsessive-compulsive disorder have persistent thoughts, impulses, or repetitive behaviors that are very stressful but which they are unable to stop by act of will. These are experienced as intrusive and senseless products of one's own mind. They are the source of much distress and interference with normal functioning.

In somatization disorder there is a history of physical complaints, including four pain symptoms, two gastrointestinal symptoms, one sexual symptom, and one pseudoneurological symptom.

Patients with dissociative fugue have sudden and temporary alterations in identity, memory, or consciousness. They may suddenly lose recollection of their past lives and a sense of who they are. These patients may leave their homes, families, and jobs and have no memory of them.

Personality Disorders, Human Sexuality, and Miscellaneous Syndromes

DIRECTIONS: Each item below contains a question or incomplete statement followed by suggested responses. Select the **one best** response to each question.

300. In narcolepsy, the polysomnographic recording typically shows

(A) an REM period shortly after sleep onset
(B) an absence of REM sleep in midcycle
(C) spike and wave EEG recording
(D) extreme muscular relaxation
(E) none of the above

301. Phobias would be LEAST likely to occur in conjunction with or as manifestations of which of the following disorders?

(A) Schizophrenia
(B) Depersonalization states
(C) Sociopathy
(D) Obsessive states
(E) Anorexia nervosa

302. A psychiatrist is traveling in Southeast Asia and is asked to consult on a young Chinese man who is terrified that his penis is shrinking and may recede into his abdomen and is convinced that this will result in death. He is certain that his condition has been caused by excessive masturbation. The most likely diagnosis is

(A) schizophrenia
(B) major depressive episode
(C) substance abuse
(D) koro
(E) amok

303. The differential diagnosis of obsessive-compulsive personality disorder includes all the following conditions EXCEPT

(A) depression
(B) anxiety disorders
(C) phobias
(D) schizophrenia
(E) impulse disorders

304. All the following are associated with narcissistic personality disorder EXCEPT

(A) intense empathy
(B) fantasies of glory
(C) entitlement
(D) exploitative behavior
(E) grandiose self-importance

305. Which of the following drugs is LEAST likely to be associated with erectile dysfunction?

(A) Benzodiazepines
(B) Antihypertensives
(C) Tricyclic antidepressants
(D) Cimetidine
(E) Neuroleptics

306. Psychogenic impotence is suggested by all the following EXCEPT

(A) sudden onset
(B) an absence of morning erections
(C) better function with some partners than with others
(D) obsession with the penis
(E) full potency with masturbation but not intercourse

307. All the following statements concerning persons with avoidant personality disorder are true EXCEPT

(A) they usually appear calm during psychiatric interviews
(B) they very much want affection and are eager to please
(C) they require uncritical acceptance before entering into a relationship
(D) in their work, they usually are on the periphery of responsibility
(E) they are hypersensitive to rejection and misinterpret social interactions

308. All the following are true statements about nocturnal penile tumescence (erection) EXCEPT

(A) it typically occurs during REM sleep
(B) it is commonly measured to assist the differential diagnosis of organic versus functional impotence
(C) its presence rules out an organic basis for male erectile disorder
(D) it is commonly combined with measurement of penile rigidity
(E) it may be affected by depression

309. An attractive and well-dressed 22-year-old woman is arrested for prostitution, but on being booked at the jail, she is found to actually be a male. The patient tells the consulting physician that he is a female trapped in a male body and has felt that way since he was a child. He has been taking female hormones and is attempting to find a surgeon who would remove his male genitals and create a vagina. The most likely diagnosis is

(A) homosexuality
(B) gender identity disorder
(C) transvestic fetishism
(D) delusional disorder
(E) schizophrenia

310. Characteristically the personality disorders

(A) are minor disturbances that respond quickly to treatment
(B) cause little impairment in adaptive functioning
(C) rarely cause any subjective distress
(D) are usually evident by adolescence
(E) often have periods of remission of up to 1 year

311. The most common finding in patients with factitious disorder is

(A) an associated major mental disorder
(B) an aggressive, assertive personality style
(C) frequent signing out of hospitals
(D) self-administered injections or self-medication
(E) lack of medical training

312. According to *DSM-IV,* the diagnosis of an adjustment disorder is limited to those patients

(A) whose symptoms are in response to an identifiable stressor that occurred within the past 2 years
(B) who do not have social impairment due to their symptoms
(C) whose symptoms are an exacerbation of a preexisting axis II disorder
(D) whose distress is in excess of what would be expected as a result of the stressor
(E) whose symptoms persist for at least 1 year after the termination of the stressor

Items 313–314

A 25-year-old man is brought reluctantly to a psychiatrist by his parents, who are concerned about his inability to hold a job. They state that since adolescence, he has been impulsive, constantly in conflict in all his interpersonal relationships, and always sees the world and himself differently than do other people. He states he does not use drugs and has no psychiatric symptoms. The mental status examination shows no cognitive deficits and no abnormality of mood, affect, or thinking.

313. The most likely diagnosis is

(A) posttraumatic stress disorder
(B) major depression
(C) schizophrenia
(D) obsessive-compulsive disorder
(E) personality disorder

314. In *DSM-IV*, the diagnosis would be recorded on axis

(A) I
(B) II
(C) III
(D) IV
(E) V

315. The capacity for female orgasm is commonly interfered with in all the following medical illnesses or treatments EXCEPT

(A) use of antidepressants
(B) use of antibiotics
(C) primary hyperprolactinemia
(D) diabetes mellitus
(E) hypothyroidism

316. Patients who have a paranoid personality disorder

(A) usually also suffer from paranoia
(B) have a predisposition to develop schizophrenia
(C) often have a preoccupation with helping the weak and the powerless
(D) usually present themselves in a quiet and humble fashion
(E) are often litigious

317. True statements about antisocial personality include all the following EXCEPT

(A) it is more frequently diagnosed in males
(B) the signs and symptoms often begin to appear in childhood
(C) common symptoms include violence and job problems
(D) it accounts for a large portion of the prison population
(E) a majority of affected persons develop serious criminality

318. A pouting and demanding 25-year-old woman begins psychotherapy stating she is both desperate and bored. She recounts a 5- or 6-year history of short episodic bursts of anxiety and depression, several theatrical suicidal gestures, impulsive and self-defeating behavior, and sexual promiscuity. She wonders if she might be a lesbian, though most of her sexual experiences have been with men. She has abruptly terminated two previous attempts at psychotherapy when she became enraged at the therapist's unwillingness to prescribe anxiolytic medication. The mental status examination shows her reality testing to be intact, and no diagnosis is apparent on axis I. The most likely axis II diagnosis is which of the following personality disorders?

(A) Paranoid
(B) Histrionic
(C) Antisocial
(D) Borderline
(E) Schizotypal

Items 319–321

A 32-year-old man comes for consultation accompanied by his wife of 10 years. The wife states that she can no longer tolerate his constant gloominess, cheerlessness, and unhappiness and also his constant brooding, complaints of inadequacy, and pessimism. He is also very negative, critical, and judgmental of others. He acknowledges that he has been this way as long as he can remember, and that it never changes. He has no complaints regarding concentration, sleep, or appetite.

319. The most likely diagnosis is

(A) avoidant personality disorder
(B) dysthymia
(C) major depressive disorder
(D) obsessive-compulsive personality disorder
(E) depressive personality disorder

320. The most common treatment for this condition is

(A) desipramine
(B) fluoxetine
(C) behavior modification
(D) family therapy
(E) psychodynamic psychotherapy

321. The most common axis I disorder associated with this condition is

(A) schizophrenia
(B) major depressive episode
(C) obsessive-compulsive disorder
(D) phobic disorder
(E) panic disorder

322. Estimates of the lifetime prevalence rates of all personality disorders in the general population range from

(A) 0.1 to 0.5 per 100
(B) 1 to 2 per 100
(C) 3 to 5 per 100
(D) 6 to 10 per 100
(E) 20 to 25 per 100

323. All the following are true statements about transvestic fetishism EXCEPT

(A) it occurs in males who are homosexual
(B) there are sexual urges and arousing fantasies associated with cross-dressing
(C) masturbation is often associated with fantasies of sexual attractiveness while dressed as a woman
(D) the disorder often begins in childhood or adolescence
(E) there is no desire for sex-reassignment surgery

324. Which of the following statements regarding vaginismus is true?

(A) It involves the outer one-third of the vagina
(B) It occurs only during attempted intercourse
(C) It is initiated by erotic arousal
(D) It makes female masturbation impossible
(E) It is under voluntary control

Items 325–326

A 40-year-old man is arrested and sent for observation after repeatedly disrupting the local IRS office with accusations that it is an arm of the Central Intelligence Agency and it is spying on him with the intent of assassination because he has relatives living in Russia. His mental status examination is unremarkable except for delusional thinking about the IRS. When his wife visits, she is found to have a somewhat passive relationship with her husband, clearly holds the same convictions that led to his arrest, and otherwise displays an unremarkable mental status.

325. The most likely diagnosis for this man's wife is

(A) paranoid schizophrenia
(B) shared psychotic disorder
(C) paranoid personality disorder
(D) obsessive-compulsive disorder
(E) avoidant personality disorder

326. If the patient's wife were to be treated, the first and most important step would be

(A) electroconvulsive therapy
(B) antidepressant medication
(C) separation from her husband
(D) family therapy
(E) behavior modification

Items 327–329

A 33-year-old married man comes for consultation because of chronic anxiety. He states his marriage is very happy and gives a sexual history that includes daily and satisfying sexual intercourse with his wife. He also masturbates three to four times weekly. He states that his sexual drive has been high ever since he was a teenager. His sexual fantasies are predominantly heterosexual, but there are occasional homosexual fantasies while masturbating. On several occasions as an adult, while traveling alone, he has had both heterosexual and homosexual experiences, which are remembered as having been pleasurable. While describing some transient guilt about "stepping out" on his wife, he is not anxious or troubled about his sexuality and does not consider it to be a problem.

327. On the basis of the patient's sexual history, one could reasonably infer a diagnosis of

(A) schizotypal personality disorder
(B) antisocial personality disorder
(C) narcissistic personality disorder
(D) borderline personality disorder
(E) no personality disorder

328. Which of the following statements is most likely to be true about the patient's masturbation and frequency of total sexual outlet?

(A) The patient has a higher-than-average sexual drive, but it is within the range of normal
(B) Regular masturbation in a married man, for whom intercourse is available, is pathologic
(C) The patient is probably hypomanic
(D) The regularity of his masturbation makes it very probable that he has falsely characterized sexuality with his wife as satisfying
(E) The patient is probably psychotic

329. Which of the following statements is most likely to be true about the history of occasional homosexual fantasies and several adult homosexual experiences?

(A) The patient is almost certainly a repressed homosexual
(B) The absence of anxiety or concern about his sexuality suggests psychopathology
(C) He may be bisexual, but nothing in the history suggests sexual psychopathology
(D) There is a need for conjoint marital therapy
(E) The patient has a disturbance of core gender identity

Items 330–331

A 35-year-old woman appears for psychiatric consultation and demands that her husband be present during the interview. He complains that he has trouble doing anything by himself because of her clinging. She at times idolizes him and, at other times, denounces him as worthless. She has a history of impulsivity with respect to spending and sexuality, and there is a conviction for reckless driving. She acknowledges chronic feelings of emptiness, fits of anger and rage when her husband "abandons" her, and lability of mood.

330. The most likely diagnosis is

(A) borderline personality disorder
(B) narcissistic personality disorder
(C) paranoid personality disorder
(D) antisocial personality disorder
(E) dependent personality

331. All the following associated features are commonly found with this disorder EXCEPT

(A) history of physical and sexual abuse
(B) history of dropping out of college just before graduation
(C) suicide attempts
(D) an absence of psychotic-like symptoms, even with stress
(E) co-occurring axis I disorder

Items 332–334

A 17-year-old high-school senior, who is 66 inches tall (168 cm) and weighs 70 lb (31.8 kg), is admitted to the hospital. She talks a great deal about her fears of "losing control" and becoming "even more fat than I am now." Despite her emaciated appearance, she diets and exercises rigorously. She insists her face, hips, and thighs are too fat. Her menstrual periods have ceased. She takes a lot of food, but eats little.

332. The most likely diagnosis is

(A) anorexia nervosa
(B) social phobia
(C) paranoid personality disorder
(D) body dysmorphic disorder
(E) major depressive disorder

333. Clinical and laboratory examination would likely reveal all the following EXCEPT

(A) bradycardia
(B) hypertension
(C) elevated serum carotene concentration
(D) hypothermia
(E) leukopenia

334. The girl described is likely to display all the following EXCEPT

(A) denial of the severity of her condition
(B) strong passive-dependent wishes
(C) features of schizophrenia
(D) depressive symptoms
(E) a need to be controlling

335. True statements about fetishism include all the following EXCEPT

(A) it occurs in both homosexuals and heterosexuals
(B) it occurs in both males and females
(C) it commonly involves an inanimate object
(D) it is frequently associated with masturbation
(E) it often exists in combination with other perversions

Personality Disorders, Human Sexuality, and Miscellaneous Syndromes

Answers

300. The answer is A. *(Hales, 2/e, pp 840–841.)* Patients with narcolepsy probably have a defect in REM inhibition, and they typically show a sleep-onset REM period or one that occurs very shortly after the onset of sleep. From 15 to 30 percent may also show some nocturnal myoclonus or sleep apnea.

301. The answer is C. *(DSM-IV, pp 409–410.)* Phobias can exist in association with schizophrenic decompensation and may be the initial manifestation of obsessions. People who have anorexia nervosa have phobic fears of losing control of their eating habits and becoming fat. Phobic attacks can be a major aspect in depersonalization states, as exemplified by the phobic anxiety-depersonalization syndrome. Phobias are not likely to be associated with sociopathic personality disorders.

302. The answer is D. *(Kaplan, 6/e, p 1056.)* These symptoms are characteristic of koro, which appears suddenly and is associated with intense fear. There are marked somatic anxiety symptoms, including palpitations, skin pallor, weakness, or fainting. The patient often clutches his penis desperately or uses strings or clamps to prevent the retraction. This condition is primarily seen in Southeast Asia, particularly among the Chinese population. Often the patient believes the problem to have been caused by sexual excesses. Sporadic cases are seen in western countries, but are usually not associated with a fear of impending death, and most often are but one manifestation of an axis I psychosis.

303. The answer is E. *(Hales, 2/e, pp 539–540.)* Obsessive-compulsive personality features can be associated with several psychiatric disorders. They can occur in depressive syndromes as well as in phobic states. An increase in obsessional thinking and compulsive behavior may herald a schizophrenic breakdown. Obsessive-compulsive people typically are cautious, controlled, and anxious, in contrast to people who have impulse disorders.

304. The answer is A. *(Hales, 2/e, pp 717–718.)* All the listed characteristics are found in narcissistic personality disorder except empathy. Patients with this disorder are notable for their lack of empathy and consideration for the feelings of others. This is associated with a grandiose sense of self-importance and a sense of entitlement. As a result their relationships tend to be self-centered and shallow.

305. The answer is A. *(Kaplan, 6/e, pp 1304–1307. Rundell, pp 473–476.)* Erectile dysfunction can occur with a wide variety of drugs, though this is more common in older men or men with underlying systemic medical illness associated with impotence. Cimetidine can interfere with androgenic receptor activity, neuroleptics can raise prolactin levels because of dopamine blockade, the tricyclic antidepressants can interfere with central serotonergic or noradrenergic pathways, and antihypertensives can also interfere with neurotransmitter systems associated with sexual functioning. Drugs of abuse such as cocaine, alcohol, morphine, and heroin are also associated with erectile dysfunction.

306. The answer is B. *(Kaplan, 6/e, pp 1304–1307.)* The psychiatric interview can often be very helpful in assisting the diagnosis of erectile dysfunction. Psychologically based dysfunction may be due to performance anxiety, psychiatric disorder, or psychodynamic conflict. Early morning erections, full function with masturbation, and better functioning with some partners all suggest a psychodynamic cause, as does a sudden rather than insidious onset of the problem.

307. The answer is A. *(Hales, 2/e, pp 718–719.)* Persons with an avoidant personality disorder are anxious, often strikingly so, during psychiatric interviews. They typically are eager to please, yet are oversensitive to perceived rejection. Despite low self-esteem and avoidance of risk, these persons desire almost desperately to be in the social and occupational mainstream. Usually, however, their relationships are distorted by their exquisite sensitivity to rejection, and they gravitate toward work roles far from the spotlight. Alliance with a therapist and assertiveness training may be quite helpful to persons who have avoidant personality disorder.

308. The answer is C. *(Hales, 2/e, p 661.)* The monitoring of nocturnal penile tumescence (NPT) is a common procedure to help differentiate organic from functional impotence. In 85 to 90 percent of cases, the presence of erections that normally accompany REM sleep will rule out a physical basis for the problem. However, men with conditions such as hyperprolactinemia or subtle vascular disorders may have erections during their REM sleep. Conversely, studies may show decreased tumescence in the absence of organic disorder; for example, in some males with depression. NPT studies are not usually necessary if the patient reports spontaneous erections, morning erections, or good erections with masturbation.

309. The answer is B. *(DSM-IV, pp 532–538.)* In adolescents and young adults, gender identity disorder is characterized by a strong cross-gender identification, a persistent discomfort with his or her sex, and clinically significant distress or impairment. Such patients usually trace their conviction to early childhood, often live as the opposite sex, and seek sex reassignment surgery and endocrine treatment. The patient feels a sense of relief and appropriateness in opposite sex clothing, in contrast to the transvestic fetishist who achieves sexual arousal from the behavior. Homosexuality is not a diagnosis in DSM-IV, and while some cross-dress to seek a same-sex partner, there is no inner conviction that they are truly of the opposite sex, nor do they seek sex reassignment surgery. These patients do not display signs of a psychotic disorder.

310. The answer is D. *(DSM-IV, pp 629–632.)* The personality disorders are deeply ingrained, inflexible patterns of perceiving, thinking about, and relating to the world. They typically result in stress and conflict in relationships as well as general impairment of adaptive functioning. The pervasive personality traits that distinguish the personality disorders are generally recognizable by adolescence or even earlier, and they typically persist throughout most of adult life.

311. The answer is D. *(DSM-IV, p 471–472. Rundell, pp 533–540.)* Patients with factitious disorder are often medical professionals or people closely associated with and knowledgeable about hospitals. Self-administered injections or ingestions of medication or foreign material (e.g., insulin, contaminants producing infection, or unacknowledged misuse of prescribed medication) are typical modes of simulating illness. These people are often passive and immature and create much controversy and anxiety in personnel who are treating them. When these patients are confronted with the diagnosis of factitious disorder, their abnormal behavior is best interpreted to them as their cry for help. Suicide attempts and signing out of hospitals are infrequent even after confrontation. These patients are not sociopathic, nor do they usually manifest psychiatric disorders.

312. The answer is D. *(DSM-IV, pp 424–429.)* According to DSM-IV, the patient's emotional or behavioral symptoms are due to a stressor that involved intense fear, helplessness, or horror with significant distress or impairment in functioning. Symptoms usually develop within 3 months of the onset of the stressor. Sometimes the onset is considerably later.

313–314. The answers are 313-E, 314-B. *(DSM-IV, pp 629–634.)* The patient displays all the features required for a diagnosis of personality disorder. These include an enduring and pervasive pattern of inner experience and behavior that deviates from the expectations of the culture in at least two of the following ways: cognition (e.g., ways of perceiving self and other people), affective responses, interpersonal functioning, and impulse control. He also meets the requirements that the problem appear by early adulthood and cause social, occupational, or other impairment. He does not show signs of psychosis, as measured by the presence of symptoms or findings on the mental status examination, nor does he demonstrate the behavioral patterns associated with posttraumatic stress disorder or obsessive-compulsive disorder.

Personality disorders and mental retardation are recorded on axis II in DSM-IV. Axis I records clinical disorders, and axis III records general medical conditions. Axis IV is used to record psychosocial and environmental problems, while axis V is used to report a global assessment of functioning (GAF).

315. The answer is B. *(Rundell, pp 468–478.)* There are a number of medical illnesses and treatments that are associated with reduced capacity for female orgasm. Diabetes mellitus, hypothyroidism, and primary hyperprolactinemia are commonly implicated. A number of drugs, such as antihypertensives and some antidepressants, may similarly interfere. Antibiotics do not commonly inhibit either male erectile function or the capacity for female orgasm.

316. The answer is E. *(Kaplan, 6/e, pp 1434–1436.)* Persons with a paranoid personality disorder characteristically show marked suspiciousness of others and are extremely sensitive to any potential threat or injustice. They frequently look for hidden motives or meanings, are contemptuous of the weak, and are very sensitive to issues of power and dominance. They often are moralistic or self-righteous and may be quite litigious. The percentage of affected persons who go on to develop schizophrenia is not known, but schizophrenia or paranoia is not the typical outcome.

317. The answer is E. *(Kaplan, 6/e, pp 1441–1444.)* Antisocial personality is diagnosed more frequently in males. Antecedent behavioral problems are usually apparent in childhood or adolescence. The most common symptoms include substance abuse, violence, and job-related, marital, and sexual problems. While antisocial personality accounts for a large portion of the prison population, only a minority of affected persons develop serious criminality. Sometimes this disorder "burns out" in middle age.

318. The answer is D. *(DSM-IV, pp 650–654.)* The history and findings are classic for the diagnosis of borderline personality disorder. These patients present with the history of a pervasive instability of mood, relationships, and self-image beginning by early adulthood. Their behavior is often impulsive and self-damaging, their sexuality is chaotic, sexual orientation may be uncertain, and anger is intense and often acted out. Recurrent suicidal gestures or behavior is common. The shifts of mood and anxiety usually last from a few hours to a few days. Patients often describe chronic feelings of boredom and emptiness.

319–321. The answers are 319-E, 320-E, 321-B. *(Kaplan, 6/e, pp 1457–1458.)* Depressive personality disorder is characterized by persistent and unremitting feelings of joylessness, dejection, and unhappiness, which date back to at least adolescence or early adulthood. There is constant worry, low self-esteem, and harsh judgment of others. Dysthymia is characterized by predominant affective and somatic symptoms rather than pervasive cognitive, interpersonal, and intrapsychic personality traits. Major depression is episodic, with predominant mood and vegetative symptoms. Persons with avoidant personality disorder are shy but not necessarily gloomy, while those with obsessive-compulsive personality are also not necessarily gloomy and tend to have restricted affective expression and to be controlling in relationships.

The most common treatment employed for patients with this diagnosis is psychodynamic psychotherapy or psychoanalysis. Such patients are generally good candidates for this treatment. Antidepressant medication is not usually employed unless there is an intervening major depression. Behavior modification might be employed to modify some specific behaviors, just as family therapy might be used to attempt to reduce interpersonal tensions. However, neither of these treatment methods would be expected to significantly alter the pervasive personality traits.

The most common associated axis I condition found in depressive personality disorder is a major depressive episode. This is typically treated with antidepressant medication. When the symptoms usually associated with depressive personality occur only during episodes of major depression, the diagnosis is not made.

322. The answer is D. *(Kaplan, 6/e, p 1431.)* Personality disorders are quite common in the general population. There is fairly good agreement that the lifetime prevalence rate of all personality disorders in the general population is about 10 percent. There is less agreement about prevalence rates for specific personality disorders largely because of sampling differences between various studies.

323. The answer is A. *(DSM-IV, pp 530–531.)* Transvestic fetishism is a condition that generally occurs in heterosexual males who experience recurrent and intensely sexually exciting urges involving cross-dressing. While cross-dressed, there is often masturbation with fantasies of sexual attractiveness while dressed as a woman. Wearing an article of women's clothing, or dressing as a woman, can also be sexually exciting while having intercourse. The condition often begins in childhood or early adolescence. Males with this disorder consider themselves to be male, but some have gender dysphoria. For diagnostic purposes the behavior must persist over a period of at least 6 months.

324. The answer is A. *(Kaplan, 6/e, pp 1310–1311.)* Vaginismus involves spasm of the musculature of the outer one-third of the vagina and thereby interferes with sexual intercourse. Usually the spasm occurs in response to any attempted penetration, including vaginal examination. Some women with this disorder are able to become excited and reach orgasm through clitoral stimulation. The vaginal muscle spasm is not under voluntary control.

325–326. The answers are 325-B, 326-C. *(DSM-IV, pp 303–304. Kaplan, 6/e, p 1044.)* Shared psychotic disorder, often called shared paranoid disorder (or folie à deux), is characterized by the transfer of delusions from the dominant personality to others in a shared and often isolated environment. Typically this involves a spouse and children. The condition is relatively rare. For the diagnosis to be made, the patient must not have had a psychotic disorder prior to adopting the induced delusion. Also, the condition must not be better accounted for by another psychotic disorder, in which case one would find the characteristic psychotic features in the mental status examination. Personality disorders are not associated with delusions.

The most important treatment is to separate the patient from the dominant partner. This provides individual support and relationship with persons who do not share the delusion. Family therapy would be contraindicated; it is not behavior that needs modification; and initial treatment would not usually involve ECT or medication.

327–329. The answers are 327-E, 328-A, 329-C. *(Kaplan, 6/e, pp 1298–1299, 1321–1333, 1425–1433.)* There is nothing in the patient's history to suggest the presence of a personality disorder. The hallmark of a personality disorder is the presence of a constellation of behaviors or traits that cause significant impairment in social or occupational functioning or cause subjective distress. There is no history of such distress or dysfunction. While some persons in our society might object to his sexual behavior on moral grounds, such judgments are not a part of the diagnostic process.

The patient gives a history of having an average of 9 to 11 orgasms per week and describes a high sexual drive since his teens. While this frequency is higher than that found in most males in their early thirties, it is neither outside the range of normalcy nor in and of itself pathologic. Similarly, the occurrence of masturbation in married men is not particularly unusual and in and of itself does not suggest a sexual disorder or marital problems. It may be due to a higher desire level than can be satisfied with his partner, it may be a relief for sexual impulses that cannot be otherwise satisfied, or it may simply be an enjoyed alternative release. Since masturbation is sometimes motivated by a desire to reduce anxiety rather than to satisfy sexual drive, it may also be related to his general anxiety. Patients who are manic or hypomanic often have increased sexual drive and frequency of release, but this tends to be episodic rather than consistent and lifelong.

Sexual behavior and fantasies range on a continuum from exclusively heterosexual to exclusively homosexual. There are many men who are predominantly heterosexual but who have engaged in homosexual behavior or have occasional homosexual fantasies, and there are many predominantly homosexual men with capacity for heterosexual arousal. The presence of homosexual desire or behavior is not considered, according to the diagnostic definitions of the American Psychiatric Association, to constitute a sexual disorder. While further therapeutic inquiry may uncover sexual conflict or marital disorder, the current history does not necessarily suggest that will be the case.

330–331. The answers are 330-A, 331-D. *(DSM-IV, pp 650–654.)* All the patient's personality traits are typical of borderline personality disorder. These patients frantically avoid real or imagined abandonment, have unstable interpersonal relations, and demonstrate impulsivity, emptiness, and inappropriate anger and affective instability. In paranoid and narcissistic personality disorder, there is a relative lack of self-destructiveness, impulsivity, and abandonment fears. Antisocial personalities are also manipulative, but they manipulate to obtain profit rather than to gain the attention of caretakers. Persons with dependent personality tend to react with appeasement and submissiveness and to seek out alternative supports when faced with fears of abandonment.

Persons with borderline personality disorder often undermine themselves when they are about to achieve a goal and typically react to stress with psychotic-like symptoms. These include transient hallucinations, distortion of body image, ideas of reference, and hypnagogic phenomena. The patient's history usually displays chaotic behavior, including suicide attempts or gestures, disrupted relationships, and a poor occupational history.

332–334. The answers are 332-A, 333-B, 334-C. *(DSM-IV, pp 539–545.)* Amenorrhea, an altered body image, and an energetic striving for thinness compose the "classic triad" associated with anorexia nervosa. The profound cachexia is not recognized in these persons, who instead strive by exercise and diet to achieve even greater thinness and to lose what they consider excess weight. In social phobia there may be embarrassment about eating in public, and in obsessive-compulsive disorder, there may be obsessions and compulsions related to food, but not the severe distortions of body image and denial of cachexia. The diagnosis of body dysmorphic disorder can be made only if the distortion is unrelated to body shape and size, for example, a preoccupation that one's eyes are too large.

These patients usually display a number of clinical and laboratory findings, including bradycardia, elevated serum carotene, leukopenia, hypothermia, and hypercholesterolemia. Hypotension, rather than hypertension, is characteristic. When the condition is associated with induced vomiting, metabolic alkalosis may ensue.

The typical patient with this condition is usually a "good child," very control oriented, and dependent. Even when warned about potential death, there is often prominent denial. Depressive symptoms are often present and may be the consequence of starvation or an underlying depression. Psychotic features are not present, as they would be in schizophrenia.

335. The answer is B. *(Kaplan, 6/e, pp 1339–1340.)* Fetishism has been reported only in males and typically involves an inanimate object that is associated with humans or their bodily adornments. It occurs in both heterosexuals and homosexuals, and often in combination with other paraphilias. Fetishism often involves masturbation, but at times it may be a part of sexual activity with a partner.

Substance-Related Disorders

DIRECTIONS: Each item below contains a question or incomplete statement followed by suggested responses. Select the **one best** response to each question.

336. All the following statements about alcoholism are true EXCEPT

(A) current classifications of alcoholic disorders are based on etiologic factors
(B) the consequences, rather than the actual amount, of drinking may be the best means for detecting alcoholism
(C) cultural background may affect the incidence of alcoholism
(D) the tendency for alcoholism to run in families is well established
(E) the reported incidence of alcoholism in women is substantially lower than in men

Items 337–339

A 50-year-old male physician with a history of meperidine (Demerol) addiction is admitted as an emergency patient for possible overdose with that drug.

337. If this is opioid intoxication, the patient can be expected to show all the following symptoms EXCEPT

(A) cyanosis
(B) hypertension
(C) drowsiness or coma
(D) slurred speech
(E) pupillary dilatation in severe overdosage

338. If the substance of intoxication was meperidine, the toxic blood level is

(A) 1 to 2 μg/dL
(B) 5 to 10 μg/dl
(C) 50 to 100 μg/dL
(D) 100 to 500 μg/dL
(E) 1000 to 2000 μg/dL

339. The treatment of opioid intoxication is commonly associated with which of the following antagonist drugs?

(A) Naloxone
(B) Haloperidol
(C) Phenobarbital
(D) Diazepam
(E) Fluoxetine

340. Another primary psychiatric illness should be seriously considered if a psychosis, precipitated by ingestion of a hallucinogen, should persist beyond

(A) 1 h
(B) 2 h
(C) 24 h
(D) 48 h
(E) 2 weeks

341. Signs of intoxication may appear when the blood alcohol level reaches

(A) 20-30 mg/dL
(B) 150-200 mg/dL
(C) 2 percent
(D) 5 percent
(E) 10 percent

342. Symptoms suggestive of schizophrenia may be seen in the abuse of all the following substances EXCEPT

(A) cocaine
(B) LSD
(C) amphetamines
(D) mescaline
(E) methaqualone

343. Death is likely to occur at a serum alcohol level of

(A) 10 to 15 mg/dL
(B) 20 to 30 mg/dL
(C) 75 to 100 mg/dL
(D) 200 mg/dL
(E) >400 mg/dL

344. All the following disturbed sexual functions are commonly found in alcoholic persons EXCEPT

(A) decreased sperm production and motility in men
(B) decreased ejaculate volume in men
(C) increased testosterone levels in men
(D) impotence
(E) menstrual irregularities in women

345. All the following statements about glue-sniffing are true EXCEPT

(A) tolerance occurs
(B) withdrawal symptoms are intense
(C) amnesia for the episode may occur
(D) it may cause irreversible damage to brain, liver, and kidney
(E) it may cause death by respiratory arrest

346. True statements about disulfiram (Antabuse) include all the following EXCEPT

(A) it interferes with the metabolic breakdown of ketones
(B) it may cause a reaction from the use of after-shave lotion
(C) it becomes fully effective only 12 h after ingestion
(D) it may cause a reaction up to 2 weeks after it is discontinued
(E) increases the blood concentration of tricyclic drugs

347. The drug of abuse 3,4-methylenedioxymethamphetamine (MDMA), often known as "ecstasy,"

(A) produces a "high" lasting 5-7 days
(B) is not associated with hallucinogenesis
(C) has a "rush" associated with an absence of sweating
(D) has little or no effects on cardiac function
(E) typically decreases sociability

348. True statements about probable genetic factors in the genesis of primary alcoholism include all the following EXCEPT

(A) the concordance for alcoholism is higher in monozygotic than in dizygotic twins
(B) children who have been separated from their alcoholic biologic parents early in life have markedly elevated rates of alcoholism
(C) the children of nonalcoholics adopted into the homes of alcoholics do not show elevated rates of alcoholism as adults
(D) there is an increased intensity of reaction to ethanol in the sons and daughters of alcoholic fathers
(E) alcoholism is probably a genetically influenced disorder with a rate of heritability similar to that expected for diabetes or peptic ulcer

Items 349–351

A 35-year-old man stumbles into the emergency room. His pulse is 100 beats per minute, his blood pressure is 170/95 mmHg, and he is diaphoretic. He is tremulous and has difficulty relating a history. He does admit to insomnia the past two nights and thinks a curtain is a ghost in the room. He also states he has been a drinker since age 19, but has not had a drink in 4 days.

349. The most likely diagnosis is

(A) adjustment disorder
(B) atypical psychosis
(C) alcohol withdrawal delirium (delirium tremens)
(D) alcohol intoxication
(E) alcohol idiosyncratic intoxication

350. Initial drug treatment usually includes

(A) haloperidol 10 mg IM
(B) chlorpromazine 50 mg IM
(C) lithium 300 mg PO
(D) chlordiazepoxide 50 mg PO
(E) imipramine 50 mg PO

351. Appropriate follow-up treatment for this patient would include all the following EXCEPT

(A) complete history and physical examination with emphasis on hepatic, gastrointestinal, and neurologic functioning
(B) psychological assessment to determine underlying psychopathology
(C) social assessment to identify social and environmental stressors
(D) referral to Alcoholics Anonymous (AA)
(E) fluphenazine decanoate (Prolixin), 1 ml IM, with an appointment to his local mental health clinic for follow-up

352. The diagnosis of alcohol dependence includes all the following EXCEPT

(A) impaired social or occupational functioning
(B) the need for daily drinking to function adequately
(C) lack of tolerance for alcohol
(D) an inability to cut down or stop drinking
(E) pathological use of alcohol

353. Adverse reactions following marijuana use include all the following EXCEPT

(A) acute panic
(B) delirium
(C) flashbacks
(D) chronic psychosis
(E) bradycardia

354. Which of the following drugs is a narcotic antagonist?

(A) Chlordiazepoxide
(B) Haloperidol (Haldol)
(C) Methadone (Dolophine)
(D) Phenobarbital
(E) Naloxone (Narcan)

355. Assay of which of the following is most apt to detect cocaine use several days earlier?

(A) Blood
(B) Hair
(C) Saliva
(D) Semen
(E) Urine

356. Physical findings commonly encountered during the examination of patients suffering from phencyclidine (PCP) intoxication include all the following EXCEPT

(A) a fixed and unwavering gaze
(B) myoclonus
(C) ataxia
(D) hypertension
(E) tachycardia

357. Abnormalities found in the offspring of women who abuse alcohol during pregnancy include all the following EXCEPT

(A) low birth weight
(B) microcephaly and maxillary hypoplasia
(C) mental retardation
(D) excessively placid and hypoactive behavior
(E) cardiac anomalies

358. A 39-year-old man enters an emergency room complaining of anxiety and extreme sleeplessness. He is noted to be markedly tremulous, and while being examined he has a grand mal seizure. This man might be suffering from withdrawal from any of the following substances EXCEPT

(A) alcohol
(B) haloperidol (Haldol)
(C) meprobamate (Equanil and Miltown)
(D) phenobarbital
(E) diazepam (Valium)

359. True statements about withdrawal from stimulants such as cocaine and amphetamines include all the following EXCEPT

(A) it may begin insidiously while the person is still taking stimulants
(B) it may include muscular aches and pains
(C) the first 9 h to 14 days are characterized by a "crash" with intense craving, agitation, depression, and insomnia
(D) following an initial acute phase of reaction, a period of fatigue, anxiety, and anhedonia occurs, which can last up to 10 weeks
(E) the usual treatment consists of weaning the patient from the drug by giving smaller and smaller doses

360. All the following drugs are used in the pharmacologic treatment of ethanol withdrawal EXCEPT

(A) benzodiazepines
(B) carbamazepine
(C) amphetamines
(D) beta-adrenergic blocking drugs
(E) antipsychotics

361. Wernicke-Korsakoff syndrome is seen in chronic alcohol abuse and is characterized by all the following symptoms EXCEPT

(A) ataxia
(B) nystagmus and paralysis of certain ocular muscles
(C) confabulation
(D) loss of remote memory
(E) confusion

362. Delirium tremens, which can develop in persons who abstain from drinking after a prolonged period of alcohol use, is characteristically associated with all the following EXCEPT

(A) bradycardia
(B) tremor
(C) vivid visual hallucinations
(D) disorientation to time and place
(E) a course of 3 to 7 days

363. There is good evidence that marijuana smoking significantly decreases one's ability to drive an automobile for up to

(A) 1 h
(B) 2 h
(C) 4 h
(D) 8 h
(E) 24 h

364. All the following are commonly used in the emergency treatment of acute toxic reaction secondary to phencyclidine (PCP) use EXCEPT

(A) alkalinization of the urine
(B) phentolamine (Regitine) drip
(C) benzodiazepines
(D) haloperidol (Haldol)
(E) gastric lavage

365. True statements about the nature and effects of caffeine include all the following EXCEPT

(A) it often worsens the symptoms of panic disorder and agoraphobia
(B) withdrawal symptoms occur with sudden cessation of chronic use
(C) flashbacks occur with toxic reactions secondary to overdose
(D) overdose is associated with anxiety, derealization, dizziness, and tinnitus
(E) the half-life of many caffeinated substances is about 3 to 7 h

Items 366–368

A 35-year-old woman has been abusing benzodiazepines, usually Valium, for at least 6 months. She uses about 40 mg/day. She is admitted to the hospital for withdrawal.

366. All the following statements about the development of potential withdrawal symptoms are true EXCEPT

(A) withdrawal is a greater risk for patients taking high doses over long periods
(B) withdrawal symptoms can occur in a patient taking benzodiazepines for 2 weeks
(C) the onset of withdrawal is earlier with agents that have a long half-life
(D) withdrawal symptoms tend to be more severe with agents that have a short half-life
(E) hospitalization is often required when usage has been at high levels over a long time

367. Typical symptoms associated with benzodiazepine withdrawal include all the following EXCEPT

(A) hypersomnia
(B) anxiety
(C) headaches
(D) tremor
(E) fatigue

368. Guidelines for the treatment of benzodiazepine discontinuance syndrome include all the following EXCEPT

(A) obtain blood and urine samples for drug and ethanol assay
(B) switch to a short-acting benzodiazepine for withdrawal
(C) stabilize the patient's dosage level
(D) reduce dosage by 30 percent on the second or third day
(E) reduce the dosage by 10 to 25 percent every few days if tolerated

DIRECTIONS: The group of questions below consists of lettered options followed by numbered items. For each numbered item, select the appropriate lettered option(s). Each lettered option may be used once, more than once, or not at all. **Choose exactly the number of options indicated following each item.**

Items 369–372

Match each description with the correct term.

(A) Tolerance
(B) Potentiation
(C) Withdrawal
(D) Dependence
(E) Addiction

369. A repertoire of behaviors that maintain drug use. **(SELECT 1 TERM)**

370. Requirement of a larger dose of the drug to obtain the same effect. **(SELECT 1 TERM)**

371. A physiologic state that follows cessation of or reduction in drug use. **(SELECT 1 TERM)**

372. A syndrome of clinically significant symptoms following cessation of substance use. **(SELECT 1 TERM)**

Substance-Related Disorders

Answers

336. The answer is A. *(Kaplan, 6/e, pp 775–777.)* Existing classifications of alcoholic disorders are predominantly descriptive; in most cases the etiology is obscure. The best means of detecting alcoholism is by being alert to the possibility in persons presenting with frequently occurring sequelae—physical, social, and psychological—of alcohol abuse. Cultural, ethnic, and social factors seem to affect prevalence rates of alcoholism; in some immigrant groups, the characteristic rate of alcoholism may persist for several generations in the United States before equaling the national norm. It is well established that alcoholism tends to run in families. More men than women still are reported to be alcoholic, but this discrepancy may reflect in part the fact that women are able to "hide" their alcohol problem with less difficulty.

337–339. The answers are 337-B, 338-D, 339-A. *(Kaplan, 6/e, pp 850, 854. Schuckit, 4/e, p 290.)* Severe opioid intoxication is associated with respiratory depression, coma, and sometimes pulmonary edema. Less severe intoxication is associated with slurred speech, psychological changes, drowsiness, and impaired memory or attention. Early on, the pupils are constricted, but with anoxia they dilate. Blood pressure is typically reduced rather than elevated.

The blood level for intoxication is 100 to 500 μg/dL. The clinician must be aware that values will vary with various laboratories. Also, symptoms may persist after blood levels return to zero.

Naloxone is an opiate antagonist used to reverse the effects of the opiate drug. The patient may need to be mechanically ventilated until the drug is given, after which one should see an increase in respiratory rate and pupillary dilatation if the pupils had been constricted.

340. The answer is E. *(Galanter, pp 152–153.)* Most cases of intoxication with a hallucinogen are over within several hours. But prolonged drug-induced psychoses may occur, especially with phencyclidine (PCP), in which the psychosis may last months. In some instances the drug appears to precipitate a latent psychotic illness, and if the psychosis persists beyond 2 weeks, this should be seriously considered.

341. The answer is A. *(Kaplan, 6/e, p 783.)* Signs of intoxication may, in some people, appear with a blood alcohol level as low as 20-30 mg/dL. Most people become significantly uncoordinated when their blood alcohol level reaches 0.1 percent. Some research has shown task impairment to begin at blood alcohol levels of about 0.5 percent. Blood alcohol level is influenced by the amount of alcohol ingested as well as by body weight.

342. The answer is E. *(Galanter, pp 181–182.)* Patients who have taken cocaine, LSD, amphetamines, or mescaline can present with clinical symptoms similar to those seen in schizophrenia. Perceptual disturbances including illusions, delusions (particularly paranoid), and hallucinations are often seen in drug abusers. Cocaine abuse may result in paranoid delusions and hallucinations somewhat similar to those seen in paranoid schizophrenia. Methaqualone belongs to the sedative-hypnotic group of drugs, and abuse is more commonly associated with disinhibition, paresthesias, and ataxia.

343. The answer is E. *(Kaplan, 6/e, p 785.)* An inexperienced drinker can show signs of intoxication at 20 to 30 mg/dL; virtually everyone is intoxicated at a level of 200 mg/dL. Above 400 mg/dL, coma or death may occur. Unconsciousness usually precedes death and may stop the individual from further drinking that would result in death.

344. The answer is C. *(Schuckit, 4/e, p 75.)* Sexual functioning is commonly disturbed in persons who abuse alcohol. Alcohol has a direct effect on the testes, which may contribute to the commonly encountered impotence and decreased sperm production and motility. Ejaculate volume is often reduced, and there is decreased production of testosterone. In women, alcohol abuse can lead to menstrual irregularities as well as to adverse effects on the developing fetus.

345. The answer is B. *(Schuckit, 4/e, p 217.)* Glue is a favorite substance of abuse in children and adolescents. Tolerance to solvents occurs rapidly, but clinically relevant withdrawal symptoms do not appear to develop. Intoxication can produce aggressive behavior, hallucinations, and amnesia for the acute period. Other volatile substances, such as toluene, lacquers, and paint thinners, are particularly dangerous because of the risk of severe tissue damage with repeated use. Death can occur by respiratory arrest.

346. The answer is A. *(Kaplan, 6/e, pp 2124–2125.)* Disulfiram (Antabuse) is sometimes used in the treatment of chronic alcoholism. It interferes with the metabolic breakdown of acetaldehyde, which is an intermediary product in the metabolism of alcohol. The resulting acetaldehyde poisoning produces very unpleasant symptoms such as headache, nausea, vomiting, and anxiety. The drug becomes fully effective about 12 h after ingestion, but is slowly excreted so that reactions with alcohol ingestion can occur as much as 2 weeks after it is discontinued. Patients must avoid all forms of alcohol, even after-shave lotions. It increases the blood concentration of a wide variety of drugs, including caffeine, diazepam, tricyclic antidepressants, and anticoagulants.

347. The answer is B. *(Schuckit, 4/e, p 192.)* MDMA ("ecstasy") is a drug that was tried in the 1970s as an adjunct to psychotherapy and later became popular as a recreational drug. It is not usually associated with hallucinations. After ingestion there is an initial phase of disorientation, followed by a "rush" that includes increased blood pressure and pulse rate, as well as sweating. Ultimately there is euphoria, and often a sense of personal enlightenment, all of which typically lasts 4 to 6 h. The drug has been associated with cardiac arrhythmia and death.

348. The answer is D. *(Schuckit, 4/e, pp 85–86.)* Adoption and other family studies have consistently supported the premise that alcoholism is a genetically influenced disorder. Most investigators believe that genetic factors place a person at a higher or lower level of vulnerability, with these genetic factors then interacting with environmental ones to give a final level of risk. Numerous studies have found that the sons and daughters of alcoholic fathers have a decreased intensity of reaction to ethanol. It is postulated that this may make it more difficult for one to perceive the internal feelings that would normally alert one to the fact it was time to stop drinking.

349–351. The answers are 349-C, 350-D, 351-E. *(Kaplan, 6/e, p 784. Schuckit, 4/e, p 102.)* Alcohol withdrawal delirium (delirium tremens) is the severest form of alcohol withdrawal. Five percent of all hospitalized alcoholics develop delirium tremens during their hospital course. Clinically, delirium tremens usually develops 2 to 7 days after cessation of drinking and is characterized by tachycardia, diaphoresis, hypertension, confusion, insomnia, illusions or visual hallucinations, and tremor. Delirium tremens is most common in people with at least a 5-year drinking history in which binges are common. Initial treatment usually involves chlordiazepoxide, 50 to 100 mg. Phenothiazines should not be used because of neurologic problems and probable preexisting hepatic impairment. Follow-up treatment should include a complete biopsychosocial evaluation. AA is an excellent referral resource.

352. The answer is C. *(Kaplan, 6/e, pp 782–783.)* Alcohol dependence involves the pathological use of alcohol that results in impaired occupational or social functioning. The alcohol-dependent person needs daily drinking to function adequately, and the pathological use is demonstrated by an inability to cut down or stop drinking despite related physical disorders, blackouts, or functional impairment. Either tolerance or withdrawal symptoms are necessary to the diagnosis. The former involves the need for increasing amounts of alcohol to achieve the desired effect, and the latter involves physical symptoms, for example, morning shaking, with reduction of drinking.

353. The answer is E. *(Schuckit, 4/e, pp 174–175.)* Anxiety or panic may occur with marijuana use. This is often precipitated by the typical tachycardia as well as the paranoid ideation that may develop. With a large dose, toxic delirium manifested by confusion, disorientation, hallucinations, delusions, and depersonalization may occur. While flashbacks are more typical with hallucinogen abuse, they may also occur with marijuana either days or weeks after the last dose. Chronic psychosis from marijuana is rare in the United States, but it has been reported in association with prolonged heavy use of very potent marijuana or hashish.

354. The answer is E. *(Kaplan, 6/e, p 856.)* Naloxone (Narcan) is an opiate antagonist. Such agents, which are not addictive, block the action of opiate compounds, thus curtailing their effects. Methadone (Dolophine) is a drug whose pharmacologic properties are similar to those of morphine. The chronic administration of methadone produces both tolerance and physical dependence. By inducing tolerance to opiate-like drugs, methadone is thought to block the euphoric effects of "street" narcotics, such as heroin.

355. The answer is E. *(Kaplan, 6/e, p 824.)* All the listed substances are used to detect cocaine use, except for semen. Blood and saliva will provide the best level of current usage, while urine assay will detect use over the preceding several days. Hair analysis can reveal the drug over weeks or months, but has little clinical applicability.

356. The answer is A. *(Galanter, pp 150–155.)* Patients with phencyclidine (PCP) intoxication usually present in a psychotic state with hallucinations and frequently violence. On examination these patients often show vertical or horizontal nystagmus, agitation, myoclonus, and ataxia. Hypertension and tachycardia are common.

357. The answer is D. *(Kaplan, 6/e, p 2220.)* The fetal alcohol syndrome (FAS) refers to one or more congenital abnormalities that occur in the offspring of women who abuse alcohol during pregnancy. These may include mental retardation, cardiac anomalies, low birth weight, and other physical abnormalities such as microcephaly, epicanthic folds, abnormal palmar creases, and short palpebral fissures. Typically these infants are irritable, tremulous, and hyperactive. They eat and sleep poorly.

358. The answer is B. *(Kaplan, 6/e, pp 618–620.)* Haloperidol (Haldol) is an antipsychotic agent of the butyrophenone class. It does not produce the classic physical dependence and withdrawal effects associated with alcohol and antianxiety agents, such as diazepam, meprobamate (Equanil and Miltown), and phenobarbital. As in the case described in the question, symptoms of withdrawal from these agents can include tremor, insomnia, and seizures.

359. The answer is E. *(Schuckit, 4/e, pp 130–132.)* Withdrawal from stimulants such as cocaine and amphetamines can be insidious or more dramatic, and the phenomenon of tolerance makes it possible for withdrawal to occur while the patient is still taking the drug. Typical symptoms during the "crash" period (9 h to 14 days) include muscular aches, intense craving, intense agitation, decreased appetite, and finally depression. After a while, fatigue and insomnia appear, the craving is decreased, and there is a sense of exhaustion. Following this phase, the next 1 to 10 weeks is associated with less depression and craving, but there is a recurrence of fatigue, anxiety, and anhedonia. A craving for the drug often persists for a long time. Treatment is abrupt withdrawal (rather than tapering), along with supportive intervention.

360. The answer is C. *(Schuckit, 4/e, pp 105–107.)* A wide variety of drugs have been used to treat the symptoms of alcohol withdrawal. The most commonly used are benzodiazepines such as diazepam (Valium) or chlordiazepoxide (Librium). Carbamazepine (Tegretol) appears to relieve most signs and symptoms of alcohol withdrawal, and beta-blockers have also been used. Amphetamines are not used.

361. The answer is D. *(Kaplan, 6/e, pp 344–345.)* Wernicke-Korsakoff syndrome is associated with chronic alcohol abuse. It results from the fact that in the presence of alcohol, thiamine is not absorbed adequately and is metabolized at a faster rate. Neurologic symptoms include ataxia, nystagmus, and paralysis of certain ocular muscles. As with all organic brain syndromes, the primary effect is a decrease in recent memory function as opposed to remote memory. Other psychological symptoms include confusion as well as confabulation to fill in memory deficits.

362. The answer is A. *(Hales, 2/e, p 370.)* Delirium tremens can occur when a person stops drinking after prolonged use of alcohol. It is a hypermetabolic state that is associated with tachycardia, fever, tremulousness, and increased blood pressure. Affected persons are confused, are disoriented to time and place, and often have visual, tactile, or olfactory hallucinations. Symptoms usually last from 3 to 7 days. The mortality is significant in untreated persons.

363. The answer is D. *(Schuckit, 4/e, pp 174–176.)* Marijuana has been clearly demonstrated to decrease judgment, impair ability to estimate time and distance, and impair motor function. As with alcohol, these effects make accidents one of the major dangers of smoking marijuana. These two substances may also potentiate each other. Up to 17 percent of drivers in fatal accidents have tested positive for cannabinols. Driving ability is significantly affected for up to 8 h after smoking, and the ability of experienced pilots to fly is significantly decreased for 24 h.

364. The answer is A. *(Schuckit, 4/e, pp 210–212.)* PCP may cause a life-threatening toxic reaction with a combination of both sympathetic and cholinergic overactivity. There are no specific antagonists to PCP, and treatment is predominantly supportive. Phentolamine is used to treat serious hypertension, and gastric lavage must be considered when the drug has been taken orally. Behavioral control is often best handled by chemical rather than physical restraint, and both haloperidol and benzodiazepines have been employed to accomplish this. Acidification of the urine to a pH less than 5.0 will decrease the half-life of PCP from 72 to 24 h. Acidification may be required for up to 2 weeks in the longer lasting toxic conditions.

365. The answer is C. *(Schuckit, 4/e, pp 251–259.)* Caffeine belongs to the xanthine group of drugs. It is capable of producing panic, anxiety, and a worsening of panic disorder and agoraphobia. The half-life of caffeine is short, and flashbacks are not encountered with this drug. Tolerance and dependence occur with chronic use, and sudden withdrawal is associated with rapid onset of headache, muscle tension, irritability, anxiety, and fatigue. Overdose can occur through excessive coffee drinking or prescription drugs containing caffeine. Symptoms of overdose include hyperstimulation, tinnitus, derealization, and even confusion and hallucinations.

366–368. The answers are 366-C, 367-A, 368-B. *(Kaplan, 6/e, pp 879–881, 883–884. Schuckit, 4/e, pp 29–30.)* Abrupt discontinuance of even therapeutic doses given over weeks (even 2 weeks) or months can result in the discontinuance syndrome. The greater the dosage and the length of time the drug has been taken, the greater the likelihood that this syndrome will occur. The onset of withdrawal is earlier with benzodiazepines that have a short half-life, and the symptoms tend to be more severe. Clinicians will often convert the patient from short to long half-life benzodiazepines, at an equivalent dosage, to achieve stabilization before withdrawal. If severe symptoms are anticipated, or when the patient is less than reliable, hospitalization is not uncommon.

Patients with the discontinuance syndrome experience symptoms involving mood, cognition, insomnia, an altered sleep-wake cycle with daytime drowsiness, and perceptual disturbances. The latter may include illusions, hallucinations, depersonalization, and blurred vision. There are also physical signs and symptoms, including tachycardia, elevated blood pressure, hyperreflexia, muscle tension, tremor, nausea, ataxia, and even grand mal seizures.

The outline for treatment begins with a thorough medical examination, including blood and urine assays. The patient is stabilized at the dosage level above that which would cause withdrawal symptoms and is often switched to a longer half-life benzodiazepine before discontinuance begins. Typically the dosage is reduced by 30 percent on the second or third day, then reduced, as tolerated, by 10 to 25 percent every few days. Detoxification from therapeutic doses is usually initiated by a 10 to 25 percent reduction, and the rate of taper is then guided by the severity of the patient's anxiety.

369–372. The answers are 369-E, 370-A, 371-C, 372-D. *(Kaplan, 6/e, pp 755, 759, 1896.)* These terms are commonly confused or used ambiguously. Tolerance refers to a pharmacologic effect in which a larger dose of a drug becomes necessary over time to achieve the same effect. Dependence is a condition in which withdrawal symptoms occur if the drug is stopped, and these symptoms indicate loss of control and usually lead to further drug use despite adverse consequences. The term addiction is often confused with dependence and refers to a whole repertoire of behaviors that serve to maintain drug use. With respect to drugs of abuse, one may see both tolerance and dependence simultaneously. The addicted person is one who has a whole series of behaviors and other phenomena that span the spectrum of the biopsychosocial structure of human existence. For this reason, successful treatment programs must be very broad in their approach to the patient's biological, psychological, and social problems.

Psychotherapies

DIRECTIONS: Each item below contains a question or incomplete statement followed by suggested responses. Select the **one best** response to each question.

Items 373–374

A 40-year-old woman, with a history of chaotic interpersonal relationships, enters psychoanalytic psychotherapy. She alternates between periods in which she idealizes the therapist and the therapy and periods of rageful anger, at which time nothing is good about the therapist or the therapy either now or in the past.

373. This is an example of the defense mechanism of

(A) reaction-formation
(B) denial
(C) projection
(D) undoing
(E) splitting

374. In which of the following diagnoses is this most commonly encountered?

(A) Schizophrenia
(B) Major depressive episode
(C) Obsessive-compulsive disorder
(D) Schizoid personality disorder
(E) Borderline personality disorder

375. In psychoanalytic theory, the phenomenon of transference

(A) occurs only in the relationship between the therapist and the patient
(B) impedes the progress of therapy because it distorts reality
(C) makes it difficult to reconstruct the patient's past
(D) involves the unconscious imposition of the experience of a past relationship onto a present one
(E) is manifested primarily in the patient's dreams

376. Therapeutic techniques commonly employed in cognitive psychotherapy include all the following EXCEPT

(A) directive statements
(B) "collaborative empiricism"
(C) behavioral techniques
(D) interpretation of dreams
(E) identification of irrational beliefs

377. True statements about hypnosis include all the following EXCEPT

(A) it is associated with an EEG pattern different from that seen in sleep
(B) in general it is a safe procedure
(C) hypnotizability increases with increasing degree of psychopathology
(D) there are tests that can indicate a person's ability to be hypnotized
(E) it is not generally appropriate for the treatment of psychotic disorders

378. Common treatments for agoraphobia include all the following EXCEPT

(A) behavior modification
(B) psychotherapy
(C) tricyclic antidepressants
(D) monoamine oxidase inhibitors
(E) electroconvulsive therapy

379. The behavioral therapy technique of systematic desensitization typically involves all the following EXCEPT

(A) homework assignments
(B) interpretation of unconscious conflict
(C) relaxation training
(D) construction of hierarchies
(E) imagined scenes

380. In the technique of behavioral therapy known as flooding, patients are exposed to what they fear

(A) in massive amounts
(B) in repeated small doses, rapidly presented
(C) in symbolic form
(D) in a relentless interpretation of their conflicts
(E) only after the fear has been neutralized by pharmacological therapy

381. According to psychoanalytic dream theory, sexual dreams involving the therapist

(A) signify the presence of severe psychopathology
(B) often express unconscious transference wishes
(C) signify a history of sexual abuse
(D) rarely occur in psychotherapy
(E) suggest a need to transfer the patient to another therapist

382. The accentuation of one side of an ambivalent pair (e.g., love-hate) in order to keep the other side in repression is known as

(A) acting out
(B) rationalization
(C) splitting
(D) sublimation
(E) reaction formation

383. The development of a transference neurosis during psychoanalytic treatment

(A) typically occurs in the final stage of analytic treatment
(B) occurs only with severely neurotic patients
(C) is therapeutically useful
(D) usually represents a repetition of rebellious adolescent conflict with authority
(E) involves negative but not positive feelings toward the analyst

384. The psychotherapy of personality disorders is made more difficult by the fact that character traits are usually

(A) ego-dystonic
(B) ego-syntonic
(C) unrelated to conflict
(D) so difficult to identify
(E) unrecognized by important persons in the patient's life

385. The time-limited psychotherapy for depression developed by Strupp and associates characteristically

(A) employs the "transference paradigm"
(B) uses hypnosis
(C) focuses exclusively on the "here and now"
(D) avoids the use of interpretation
(E) includes behavioral deconditioning exercises

386. Otto Kernberg's theories about the diagnosis and treatment of borderline personality emphasize the crucial importance of the defense mechanism of

(A) splitting
(B) sublimation
(C) isolation
(D) somatization
(E) suppression

387. All the following are true statements about supportive psychotherapy EXCEPT

(A) regressive transference is encouraged and interpreted
(B) it is generally used for healthy persons in crisis or for patients with ego deficits
(C) a major goal is to support reality testing
(D) suggestion and reassurance are employed
(E) there is an attempt to strengthen defenses

388. In psychoanalytic psychotherapy the occurrence of countertransference is

(A) inevitable to the process
(B) almost always harmful to the process
(C) a sign that the patient should be referred to another therapist
(D) a sign that the therapist is excessively neurotic
(E) an indication that the therapist dislikes the patient

389. Client-centered psychotherapy stresses which of the following characteristics in the therapist?

(A) Unconditional positive regard for the patient
(B) Intellectual reasoning power
(C) Confrontational ability
(D) Sensitivity to unconscious conflict
(E) Ability to give reality-based advice

390. Erik Erikson's concept of the life cycle is characterized by all the following EXCEPT

(A) eight states of ego development
(B) the epigenetic principle
(C) phase-specific developmental crisis
(D) personality development completed by the end of adolescence
(E) generativity

391. Cognitive psychotherapy tends to focus heavily on

(A) unconscious and repressed memories
(B) mistaken ideas and beliefs
(C) transference ideation
(D) projective identifications
(E) none of the above

392. The form of psychoanalytic intervention developed by Heinz Kohut stresses

(A) confrontation
(B) interpretation of resistance and defense
(C) developmental conflict
(D) developmental deficit
(E) cognitive development

393. A 25-year-old man seeks psychiatric consultation because of anxiety, conflict with his new wife, and a chaotic work history. Examination reveals the presence of an underlying paranoid personality. Psychotherapy is suggested as part of the recommended treatment. Which of the following therapies is most likely to be CONTRAINDICATED?

(A) Hypnosis
(B) Cognitive therapy
(C) Family therapy
(D) Supportive psychotherapy
(E) Psychodynamic psychotherapy

394. To be treated successfully in psychoanalysis, a neurotic patient must have all the following attributes EXCEPT

(A) a reservoir of basic trust
(B) a capacity for reality testing
(C) a capacity for internalization
(D) an ability to tolerate a dependent position
(E) age of at least 21

395. Which of the following statements is true of the psychoanalytic psychotherapy of patients with severe oedipal conflicts?

(A) The therapist should be of the same sex as the patient
(B) The therapist should be a male if the patient is female
(C) The development of an intense transference should be avoided
(D) The therapist should de-emphasize sexual topics
(E) None of the above

396. All the following statements about interpersonal psychotherapy (IPT) for depression are true EXCEPT

(A) it is a brief, weekly psychotherapy
(B) it was developed for ambulatory, nonbipolar, nonpsychotic patients
(C) the focus is mainly on current problems, conflicts, wishes, and frustrations
(D) regressive transferences are encouraged and interpreted
(E) rational problem solving is stressed

397. Traditional psychoanalysis is commonly used in the treatment of persons affected by all the following conditions EXCEPT

(A) conversion disorders
(B) obsessive-compulsive disorders
(C) personality disorders
(D) psychotic disorders
(E) certain perversions

398. Interpersonal psychotherapy (IPT), as developed by Klerman and his colleagues, is accurately characterized by all the following statements EXCEPT

(A) it would be useful in treating self-defeating patterns of relationships
(B) it is often combined with medication
(C) it was developed to treat patients with nonpsychotic major depression
(D) the primary emphasis is on conjoint treatment of couples and group psychotherapy
(E) it aims to improve interpersonal communication

399. An appropriate therapeutic attitude toward the schizophrenic patient includes all the following EXCEPT

(A) respect for the patient's need for privacy
(B) a consistent approach to the patient
(C) a desire to rescue the patient
(D) a focus on the patient's assets as well as on the patient's pathology
(E) tolerance of negative or bizarre behaviors

400. In general, group therapy is intended to enable individuals to do all the following EXCEPT

(A) learn new models of behavior
(B) discover that their problems are not unique
(C) develop a sense of belonging
(D) develop "basic trust"
(E) change their behavior to comply with group models

401. A patient in psychoanalysis is always anxious to please. However, he states that he has recently begun to feel frightened in the presence of the analyst and is having fantasies that he will be attacked. After listening to the patient's associations, the analyst indicates that his passive and compliant relationship with his idealized father may have been a reaction to fears that his father would hurt him.

This is an example of

(A) confrontation
(B) interpretation
(C) clarification
(D) desensitization
(E) flooding

402. A 29-year-old graduate student in molecular biology comes to his psychoanalysis tearful and angry because his major professor banished him from his laboratory, stating that he could no longer tolerate the patient's frequent critical and angry outbursts. The patient is anguished at the anticipated reaction of his father, who is a professor of molecular biology at another university. Were the therapist to respond by remarking how painful this must be for the patient, especially since his father had always been similarly rejecting, this would be particularly characteristic of which of the following theories of psychoanalytic treatment?

(A) Self-psychology
(B) Classical psychoanalysis
(C) Kleinian psychoanalysis
(D) Ego psychology
(E) Fairbairnian psychoanalysis

403. The developmental theories of John Bowlby stress

(A) aggression
(B) attachment
(C) instinctual conflict
(D) punitive superego
(E) empathy

404. Hypnotizability is primarily related to

(A) gullibility
(B) compliance
(C) suggestibility
(D) passivity
(E) conformity

405. A 49-year-old man with hypertension and anxiety is attached to an apparatus that measures skin temperature and emits a tone proportional in loudness to the temperature. This is an example of a therapeutic technique called

(A) hypnosis
(B) behavior modification
(C) supportive psychotherapy
(D) placebo therapy
(E) biofeedback

406. A 16-year-old boy is hospitalized on the adolescent ward of a mental hospital. He consistently avoids bathing and personal hygiene and is resistant to changing his behavior. A system is established wherein the patient earns "points" for accomplishing various aspects of personal hygiene. Points can be redeemed at the snack shop, or they can "purchase" extra activity passes. This is an example of a treatment method called

(A) token economy
(B) social skills training
(C) authoritarian psychotherapy
(D) self-psychology
(E) cognitive remediation

407. In most sex therapies, treatment of premature ejaculation involves all the following techniques EXCEPT

(A) cognitive re-education
(B) sensate focus
(C) stop-start technique
(D) squeeze technique
(E) use of anesthetic ointments

408. Placebos have been shown to be

(A) frequently effective in the treatment of schizophrenia
(B) frequently effective in the treatment of paranoid psychosis
(C) ineffective in relieving neurotic symptoms
(D) capable of producing significant side effects
(E) ineffective in assisting social rehabilitation in formerly psychotic patients

409. The family of a hospitalized and acutely schizophrenic patient have insisted that they want the patient treated by psychotherapy and not with drugs. All the following are true statements that could be made by the attending psychiatrist EXCEPT

(A) antipsychotic medication can rapidly relieve psychotic symptoms
(B) in preventing relapse, psychotherapy combined with antipsychotic medication is no more effective than antipsychotic medication alone
(C) psychotherapy alone usually has little effect on acute psychotic symptoms
(D) psychotherapy can be effective in assisting social rehabilitation
(E) psychotherapy alone can have an adverse effect on some schizophrenic patients

410. Existential psychotherapy is chiefly characterized by

(A) emphasis on psychopathology
(B) lack of emphasis on personal meaning
(C) emphasis on past developmental conflict
(D) lack of emphasis on spirituality
(E) individual responsibility for one's own self-definition and nature

411. Following inpatient hospitalization for an acute psychotic disorder, a 22-year-old woman is discharged to a day hospital. Partial hospitalization offers all the following services or advantages over outpatient treatment EXCEPT

(A) it diminishes isolation and dependency
(B) it provides a highly formalized medical setting that promotes security
(C) it provides much more therapeutic contact than does individual outpatient treatment
(D) it provides a therapeutic social milieu
(E) it allows greater opportunities for social and vocational rehabilitation

412. A 45-year-old woman consults a psychiatrist because of fearfulness about potential violence by her husband. In obtaining a history, all the factors below have an association with increased risk for violence EXCEPT

(A) alcohol use
(B) a history of child abuse
(C) low socioeconomic status
(D) antisocial personality disorder
(E) high levels of 5-hydroxyindoleacetic acid (5-HIAA) in cerebrospinal fluid

413. According to the cognitive model of depression, the majority of depressed patients exhibit all the following characteristics EXCEPT

(A) a chronically negative view of the self
(B) life experience interpreted in a predominantly negative way
(C) a view of the future that is pessimistic
(D) unconscious conflict regarding the aggressive drive
(E) symptoms and affects derived from negative cognitive schema

414. All the following techniques are used in the treatment of female orgasmic disorder EXCEPT

(A) prohibition of masturbation
(B) re-education about female sexuality and orgasm
(C) sensate focus exercises
(D) exercising of the pubococcygeus muscle
(E) couples therapy

415. A 34-year-old mathematician is in psychoanalytic psychotherapy because of anxiety, depression, and marital problems, which seemed to begin shortly after the death of his mother. They had an intensely dependent and ambivalent relationship with each other. When the patient discusses his mother and her death, it is intellectual, with detachment and an absence of affect. This is an example of

(A) projection
(B) isolation
(C) splitting
(D) reaction-formation
(E) projective-identification

DIRECTIONS: The group of questions below consists of lettered options followed by numbered items. For each numbered item, select the appropriate lettered option(s). Each lettered option may be used once, more than once, or not at all. **Choose exactly the number of options indicated following each item.**

Items 416–419

For each patient, select the most appropriate therapeutic option.

(A) Psychoanalysis
(B) Brief individual psychotherapy
(C) Community meeting
(D) Behavior therapy
(E) Family therapy

416. A young woman with no previous psychiatric history develops an incapacitating fear of driving after being involved in a minor automobile accident.
(SELECT 1 THERAPEUTIC INTERVENTION)

417. A 40-year-old married man, a successful businessman with a satisfying family life, is preoccupied with thoughts of becoming involved with a younger woman. He has no prior psychiatric history and no other complaints.
(SELECT 1 THERAPEUTIC INTERVENTION)

418. A 16-year-old girl begins acting out sexually. Her school performance deteriorates. These symptoms coincide with the onset of frequent arguments between her parents, who have been threatening marital separation.
(SELECT 1 THERAPEUTIC INTERVENTION)

419. An intelligent 25-year-old single woman, who has a successful career, complains of multiple failed relationships with men, unhappiness, and a wish "to sort out my life." A previous experience in individual psychotherapy had been somewhat helpful. **(SELECT 1 THERAPEUTIC INTERVENTION)**

Psychotherapies

Answers

373–374. The answers are 373-E, 374-E. *(Hales, 2/e, pp 156–160.)* This is a classic example of the defense mechanism known as splitting. Rather than an integrated ambivalence that recognizes both good and bad aspects of the other person, the person is seen as either all good or all bad.

This defense mechanism is particularly seen in patients with a borderline personality disorder. They respond to frustration or rejection with anger and devaluation, during which time the previous "good aspects" of the therapist or therapy are forgotten. This mechanism leads to chaotic interpersonal relationships.

375. The answer is D. *(Nersessian, pp 419, 430–432.)* Transference is a ubiquitous phenomenon, but it is especially prominent in psychoanalytic therapies because they are conducted so as to maximize its occurrence. The discovery of transference by Sigmund Freud was one of his most important contributions. Transference involves the patient's seeing and experiencing the present through "past-colored glasses," thereby making it possible to reconstruct the past and understand the origin of the patient's conflicts. While it certainly may color the patient's dreams, its predominant manifestations are in the interactions with the therapist or analyst in the course of treatment.

376. The answer is D. *(Andreasen, 2/e, pp 635–638.)* Cognitive psychotherapy is a directive and time-limited psychotherapy that does not involve itself with the unconscious and therefore dream interpretation. It aims to identify and eliminate negatively biased thinking and to foster greater logical and reality-based thinking. It was originally developed with nonpsychotic depressed patients, but is now used in a wide variety of conditions. "Collaborative empiricism" refers to the collaboration between therapist and patient to identify the patient's irrational beliefs and illogical thinking patterns. The treatment is structured and behavioral.

377. The answer is C. *(Kaplan, 6/e, p 1807.)* The hypnotic state is not identical to sleep, and sleep EEG patterns are not seen. The neurophysiology of the trance state is not well understood. While there is considerable controversy about the clinical usefulness of hypnosis in psychotherapy, it is a safe procedure when used in a professional manner. There are numerous tests of hypnotizability, and the ability to be hypnotized is not related to the degree of psychopathology. It is generally not employed with psychotic patients.

378. The answer is E. *(Andreasen, 2/e, pp 302–303.)* The most common treatment for agoraphobia combines drugs with behavior modification or psychotherapy or both. Drugs that have proved to be particularly useful include the tricyclic antidepressants, the monoamine oxidase inhibitors, benzodiazepines such as alprazolam, and serotonin reuptake inhibitors (SRI). The psychotherapy techniques are generally targeted toward helping the patient reenter phobic situations and deconditioning their anticipatory anxiety and avoidance.

379. The answer is B. *(Hales, 2/e, pp 1062–1063.)* The behavioral technique of systematic desensitization is typically used to treat patients who have learned (conditioned) emotional reactions, for example, fears and phobias. The patient is taught relaxation, and a hierarchy of increasingly fearful images or situations is constructed. Often using imagined scenes, the patient proceeds up the hierarchy from the least feared to the most feared, learning to substitute relaxation for the previously anxious response. Exploring the unconscious and interpreting unconscious conflict are not a part of this type of treatment.

380. The answer is A. *(Hales, 2/e, p 1063.)* In flooding, patients are exposed to whatever produces their fear in as massive a quantity and for as long a duration as can be tolerated. Ultimately the fear response begins to dampen, until the patient can no longer feel it. The stimuli can be imaginary, or an in vivo exposure can be produced. This is a form of desensitization.

381. The answer is B. *(Nersessian, pp 23–26.)* Psychoanalytic dream theory views dreams as distorted, disguised, and condensed expressions of the dreamer's unconscious wishes. Dreams often express the unfolding of transference feelings or a transference neurosis and may involve a wide variety of wishes and feelings, including sexual ones. There is no implication with such dreams that the patient has severe psychopathology, a history of abuse, or is in need of transfer to a new therapist.

382. The answer is E. *(Hales, 2/e, pp 156–160.)* In reaction formation, the person deals with emotional conflict or with internal or external stressors by substituting behavior or feelings that are diametrically opposed to his or her unacceptable thoughts or feelings. Often this takes place unconsciously. The other mentioned defenses involve different mechanisms. In acting out, there is behavior without regard for negative consequences, and rationalization involves self-serving but incorrect explanations. In splitting, persons view themselves or others as either all good or all bad. It represents a failure to integrate both positive and negative qualities. Sublimation has to do with channeling unacceptable feelings or impulses into socially desirable behavior.

383. The answer is C. *(Nersessian, pp 432–435.)* The transference neurosis typically occurs during the middle stage of analytic treatment and is associated with the patient's experiencing a psychological regression to earlier developmental times of conflict. Because of the transference, patients experience what is in essence a "substitute neurosis" in which their earlier wishes and conflicts are experienced vis-a-vis the analyst. This is therapeutically useful because it helps to bring forth important memories, feelings, and reactions that can be interpreted and ultimately resolved in the context of the relationship with the analyst.

384. The answer is B. *(Kaplan, 6/e, p 466.)* In the personality disorders, character traits are typically ego-syntonic. This means they usually cause the patient little personal distress, which makes motivation for change less likely. This is in contrast to neurotic symptoms, which are experienced as unwanted "foreign bodies." The patient's character traits often cause great distress to those who must live with them. Character traits are formed in response to developmental relationships and conflict, as are neurotic symptoms. They become part of the patient's style of living and relating to others.

385. The answer is A. *(Hales, 2/e, pp 1012–1018.)* A number of brief dynamic psychotherapies have been developed for the treatment of depression. The treatment proposed by Strupp is consistent with psychoanalytic theory and is distinguished especially by its focus on the therapeutic relationships and the "transference paradigm." Strupp and associates believe that this is the best way to uncover and correct the early conflicts and maladaptive patterns that make the patient vulnerable to depression. Interpretation is an important part of this process.

386. The answer is A. *(Kaplan, 6/e, p 1440.)* Kernberg emphasized the crucial importance of splitting in the diagnosis and treatment of borderline personality disorder. Splitting involves a failure to integrate the good and bad qualities of self and others into cohesive images, which often results in the same person's being alternately idealized/loved and devalued/hated. This prevents the patient from diffusing anxiety and maintaining stable and positive introjects. Other defense mechanisms also have importance but tend to be subsidiary to this process.

387. The answer is A. *(Andreasen, 2/e, pp 642–643.)* Supportive psychotherapy is generally employed for crisis intervention and with patients whose ego-deficits or life circumstances make other forms of therapy inappropriate or impractical. The therapist attempts to maintain a reality-based, problem-solving, concerned relationship that will augment the patient's ego strengths and defenses. Commonly this will include giving advice, reassurance, and suggestion and assisting in reality testing. The treatment is not structured to maximize the likelihood of transference distortions as, for example, in psychoanalytic psychotherapy. Regression would not be encouraged, either in the transference or in general behavior.

388. The answer is A. *(Nersessian, pp 438–439, 474–476.)* Countertransference refers to unconscious needs, wishes, or conflicts in the analyst that are evoked by the patient. These reactions might result in either positive or negative feelings about or responses to the patient. Countertransference has a definite potential to be harmful to treatment by interfering with objective judgment and reason. However, it is inevitably present in psychoanalysis and probably all forms of treatment. Often it serves the very positive function of alerting the analyst to subtle or covert patient behaviors or of helping to provide insight into the patient's behavior and feelings. The only instance in which referral to another analyst is indicated would be when the first analyst is unable to resolve a countertransference that is an impediment to treatment.

389. The answer is A. *(Kaplan, 6/e, pp 1866–1868.)* Client-centered therapy was developed by the psychologist Carl Rogers. It was initially known as "nondirective" psychotherapy. It is based on the belief that people have great capacity for self-understanding and constructive emotional growth, which can be realized in the context of a special kind of relationship. This relationship is characterized by a nonjudgmental attitude, caring, empathy, and unconditional positive regard.

390. The answer is D. *(Hales, 2/e, pp 167–168.)* Erikson postulates that the life cycle consists of eight stages of ego development that commence with birth and end with death. The stages are based on the principle of epigenesis. Like the human embryo, personality development follows a predetermined sequence of steps governed by inner laws of development. Each developmental stage is characterized by a specific conflict during which opposing psychosocial attitudes vie for ascendancy. This creates a specific developmental crisis, the resolution of which allows each person to move on to the next developmental stage. Unlike Freud, who was primarily concerned with childhood psychosexual development, Erikson believes that personality develops throughout life. Generativity refers to central tasks of Erikson's stage of adulthood. These include caring for, and training, the next generation, betterment of society, and the production of ideas through one's work.

391. The answer is B. *(Hales, 2/e, pp 1084–1086.)* Cognitive therapy is usually an active, structured, time-limited form of therapy. It is based on the premise that the way we process information and structure our experiences determines how we think and feel. The patient is helped to identify, test the reality of, and correct distorted and dysfunctional beliefs that distort cognitions. This leads to more realistic and adaptive information processing and, therefore, improvements in symptoms and behavior.

392. The answer is D. *(Kaplan, 6/e, pp 460–463.)* Heinz Kohut began his career as a Freudian psychoanalyst, but later departed from classical theory to found what is sometimes known as "self-psychology." He was less concerned with resistance, defense, and conflict than he was with developmental deficits that left lasting scars in the areas of self-cohesion and self-esteem. Important among these deficits were failures in such things as empathy and mirroring by which a child develops a sense of worth.

393. The answer is A. *(Kaplan, 6/e, p 1818.)* Hypnosis has been used to treat a wide variety of psychiatric conditions and a wide variety of symptoms. However, it is not employed in the treatment of psychotic patients, and it is generally contraindicated in paranoid patients. Such patients tend to incorporate the hypnosis into their paranoid systems.

394. The answer is E. *(Kaplan, 6/e, pp 468–469. Nersessian, pp 450-453.)* Criteria for the analyzability of a person's neurosis include all the following: the ability to test reality; a sense of trust in the therapist as well as in oneself to face unpleasant issues; the ability to tolerate dependence; the capacity to internalize experience; and the motivation to pursue an unknown course. Although the above qualities suggest the presence of a certain degree of maturity, analysis can be undertaken in adolescence.

395. The answer is E. *(Nersessian, pp 432–435.)* There is nothing about oedipal conflict that in and of itself would dictate the need for a therapist of the same or opposite sex. The patient will experience a transference independent of the sex of the analyst, for example, a mother-transference to a male analyst. Since psychoanalytic psychotherapy uses transference as a major vehicle to both uncover and then resolve conflict, one would certainly not discourage the development of transference. Similarly, it would not further the therapeutic work to de-emphasize sexual topics since they are important to oedipal conflict and therefore its resolution.

396. The answer is D. *(Andreasen, 2/e, pp 641–642.)* Interpersonal psychotherapy (IPT) was developed for the brief (generally 12 to 16 weeks) treatment of ambulatory, nonpsychotic, depressed patients. It is based on the premise that interpersonal problems are commonly associated with acute depression. The focus of the treatment is mostly on the here and now, with less attention paid to early developmental considerations. The therapeutic relationship is structured as an active collaboration.

397. The answer is D. *(Kaplan, 6/e, pp 468–469.)* Psychoanalysis is a commonly used treatment for persons who have long-standing neurotic problems or character disorders. These problems include conversion disorders, phobias, obsessive-compulsive neuroses, and certain perversions. Generally, persons who are psychotic or addicted to drugs or alcohol have underlying pathology too severe to withstand the demands of analysis. There are, of course, exceptions.

398. The answer is D. *(Kaplan, 6/e, pp 1879–1880.)* Interpersonal psychotherapy is a brief treatment focusing on interpersonal problems and was developed for patients with nonpsychotic major depression. It is an individual psychotherapy aiming to improve communication and reality testing, clarify feeling states, and facilitate interpersonal skills. It is usually combined with antidepressant medication. While the treatment is based on psychodynamic theory, the focus is on current interpersonal events rather than intrapsychic issues. Examples would be role disputes, role transitions, and interpersonal deficits such as self-defeating patterns of relationships.

399. The answer is C. *(Kaplan, 6/e, pp 1009–1013.)* Therapists' attitudes toward the schizophrenic patient are a central aspect of therapeutic technique. If therapists feel they must rescue the schizophrenic patient, negative therapeutic reactions may result. Therapists should be more concerned with being of use to those patients. Important aspects of therapists' attitudes include their consistency and availability; respect for the patient; valuing the patient's autonomy; an ability to focus on the patient's assets; tolerance for negative, bizarre, and incomprehensible behavior; and therapeutic optimism.

400. The answer is D. *(Kaplan, 6/e, pp 1821–1829.)* Many processes important to group therapy have been described. Cohesion is a fundamental process by which members develop a sense of belonging or loyalty. The group may draw on an individual's desire to "belong" when it exerts group pressure to initiate change in the individual. The group also provides a variety of models of behavior that group members may imitate. By universalization, a phenomenon common to groups, members learn that others have problems similar to their own. The goal is not to suppress individuality but to help the patient understand how his or her individuality affects others, and vice versa. Primitive defects in "basic trust" are usually not appropriately treated by group psychotherapy.

401. The answer is B. *(Hales, 2/e, p 161.)* Interpretation involves the analyst's making connections and meaning out of what is happening in the analysis. These interpretations have the intent of linking the historical past to the present, often allowing unconscious memories to become conscious. The example here is of interpretation of the transference, though it is likely to help explain the patient's behavior in other interpersonal relationships.

402. The answer is A. *(Kaplan, 6/e, pp 163–164.)* Self-psychology stresses the importance of empathic response in an effort to correct empathic deficiencies in the patient's development. In this instance, the analyst's empathic response is in contrast to that of the patient's father and the major professor. Classical psychoanalysts might be more apt to focus on the patient's ambivalence about his father and how his provocative behavior with the professor related to those unresolved conflicts.

403. The answer is B. *(Kaplan, 6/e, p 167.)* John Bowlby, an English psychoanalyst, was particularly oriented toward a developmental theory that stresses the importance of early attachment behavior. He elaborated five responses associated with attachment behavior: sucking, clinging, following, crying, and smiling. He believed that the way these elements played out in early child development influenced ultimate cognitive functions and character structure.

404. The answer is C. *(Kaplan, 6/e, pp 809–810.)* Hypnotizability is primarily related to the patient's responsiveness to suggestion for altering his subjective experience. One can determine hypnotizability by using standard tests of responsiveness to suggestion. This is a more important factor than the skill of the hypnotist.

405. The answer is E. *(Kaplan, 6/e, p 1803.)* This is an example of biofeedback, used in an attempt to induce relaxation and thereby peripheral vasodilatation, which in turn lowers blood pressure. The peripheral dilatation increases skin temperature, and the audible tone helps the patient learn what he needs to do to achieve that elevation. Some clinicians feel that simple relaxation training can accomplish the same goal.

406. The answer is A. *(Kaplan, 6/e, p 2710.)* Using points, tokens, or credits to reinforce desired behaviors and token "fines" to discourage undesirable behavior is called a token economy. It may be used to reinforce social skills training or participation in therapeutic activities. To be effective, the entire staff must be united and consistent in providing positive and negative consequences for target behaviors.

407. The answer is E. *(Hales, 2/e, pp 664–665.)* The treatment of premature ejaculation has a high success rate. The treatment usually involves both partners, who are educated to understand the nature of the problem prior to beginning sensate focus. This is a series of exercises designed to increase awareness of pleasurable sensations of touch, sound, and sight. The "squeeze technique" is an exercise in which the penis is stimulated to the first sensations of impending orgasm, then strongly squeezed at the coronal ridge, which causes detumescence. The stop-start technique consists of stimulating the man to a point just short of inevitable orgasm; at that point, stimulation is halted until the sensation of impending orgasm subsides. The use of anesthetic ointments has proved unsatisfactory in treatment of premature ejaculation.

408. The answer is D. *(Kaplan, 6/e, pp 1266–1267, 2146.)* A placebo is a pharmacologically inert substance that the user believes to be a potent drug. Placebos have been shown to relieve a variety of neurotic symptoms, including anxiety and depression. They often produce side effects, such as weakness, headache, and gastrointestinal symptoms. Placebo effects are influenced by the attitudes and expectations of both physician and patient. Primary schizophrenia and psychotic reactions do not respond to placebos, but placebos may assist social rehabilitation in formerly psychotic patients.

409. The answer is B. *(Kaplan, 6/e, pp 900–901.)* Psychotherapy alone has been found to be less effective than drug treatment alone and does little to resolve acute psychotic symptoms. However, when drug treatment is combined with psychotherapy, there is greater protection from recurrence of the psychotic symptoms. Some acutely ill schizophrenic patients have an adverse response to attempts at psychotherapy, but it can be of help later during social rehabilitation.

410. The answer is E. *(Kaplan, 6/e, p 1822.)* Existential psychotherapy departs from traditional psychotherapy in that emphasis is placed on a person's own sense of meaning of his or her life rather than on psychopathology or past development. Spiritual values are also important in existential psychotherapy. Exponents of this view suggest that each individual determines his or her own nature by a constant act of self-definition for which the individual is solely responsible.

411. The answer is B. *(Kaplan, 6/e, p 2693.)* Partial hospitalization provides a therapeutic community that is transitional between the hospital and community living or as an alternative to hospitalization. The patient is in contact with a therapeutic setting for many more hours and has a wider variety of approaches to treatment and rehabilitation than is provided by outpatient treatment. The atmosphere of most day hospitals is an informal or clublike one that facilitates social interaction as well as therapeutic and rehabilitative activities. An important advantage of partial hospitalization is that it diminishes dependency as well as social isolation.

412. The answer is E. *(Andreasen, 2/e, pp 521–522.)* Patients who abuse alcohol or other substances are more likely to be violent because it causes disinhibition. Patients with schizophrenia, mania, mental retardation, brain disorder, and antisocial personality are more likely to be violent than other psychiatric patients. A history of child abuse increases the risk for violence, as does low socioeconomic status. Low, rather than high, levels of 5-HIAA have been associated with increased risk of violence, and it is hypothesized that this is because it may be a marker for impulsivity.

413. The answer is D. *(Kaplan, 6/e, pp 1183–1185.)* Cognitive theorists relate the development of psychiatric symptoms and syndromes to habitual errors in thinking (cognition). The depressed person is viewed as one whose symptoms and affects are the logical outcome of negative cognitive patterns. Self, experience, and future are viewed through "negative colored glasses." Cognitive patterns are developed early in life and may be activated or accentuated by life situations or stress.

414. The answer is A. *(Hales, 2/e, pp 663–664.)* Treatment usually begins with a thorough medical and psychiatric evaluation, a careful sexual history, and re-education regarding female sexuality and orgasm. Couples therapy may be employed when it is believed that problems in the relationship are involved in the patient's anorgasmia. The patient is instructed in sensate focus exercises to increase her awareness and comfort with bodily pleasure and is also instructed to exercise the pubococcygeus muscle. She is then instructed in a masturbatory program, which begins with body stimulation gradually proceeding to genital stimulation. Fantasy is encouraged, and once the woman is able to achieve orgasm with self-stimulation, she then teaches her partner the type of genital stimulation she requires for orgasm.

415. The answer is B. *(Andreasen, 2/e, p 645.)* Isolation is a defense mechanism for coping with intense emotions. The feelings are stripped away, and what is left is an intellectual and detached discussion of the topic associated with intense emotion. Often the patient will be overly abstract and will have difficulty in recalling or describing past feelings as well. This defense is often found in patients with obsessive-compulsive traits.

416–419. The answers are 416-D, 417-B, 418-E, 419-A. *(Andreasen, 2/e, pp 632-633. Kaplan, 6/e, pp 1042, 1873–1881. Hales, 2/e, pp 1177–1185, 1236.)* Systematic desensitization, which is a form of behavior therapy, is the most appropriate treatment for this woman. Systematic desensitization is used to treat classic phobias, but this technique as well as other forms of behavior therapy may also be of benefit in the treatment of other psychiatric disorders. It would be expected to be a good choice of treatment since the phobia appears not to be associated with other complicating psychiatric problems.

Patient selection is an important aspect of brief psychotherapy. Using psychoanalytic principles, the clinician attempts to select patients who are above average in intelligence, motivated, and able to think psychologically. Having a focused chief complaint, e.g., this man's interest in a younger woman, is also crucial. Given this man's good work history, family life, lack of previous psychotherapy, and focused complaint, brief psychotherapy is a suitable treatment. Were it to uncover other, significant problem areas, then a longer term therapy might be indicated.

Family therapy is a treatment of choice because this girl's symptomatic behavior appears to be linked to her parents' marital difficulties. Individual treatment, which would address the symptoms of the girl described in item 418, would not alter the marital or family problems, nor would it allow the parents to explore the impact of their daughter's symptoms on the marital relationship.

The woman described in item 419 is likely to be an appropriate candidate for psychoanalysis. She describes long-standing problems in heterosexual relationships. These are likely to be due to unconscious conflicts. In addition, she is unhappy with her life. Because previous psychotherapy helped but did not stop her symptoms, assessment for psychoanalysis is a reasonable therapeutic intervention.

Psychopharmacology and Other Therapies

DIRECTIONS: Each item below contains a question or incomplete statement followed by suggested responses. Select the **one best** response to each question.

420. A 35-year-old woman has a diagnosis of chronic schizophrenia. All the following drugs would commonly be considered as possible medications to control her psychotic symptoms EXCEPT

(A) haloperidol (Haldol)
(B) chlorpromazine (Thorazine)
(C) risperidone (Risperdal)
(D) olanzapine (Zyprexa)
(E) lithium

421. Because of a psychotic illness, a young man is started on high-potency neuroleptic medication and shortly thereafter develops pacing, an inability to sit still, and restless leg symptoms, which lead to the diagnosis of akathisia. The medication most likely to prove helpful is

(A) barbiturate
(B) propranolol
(C) phenytoin
(D) a neuroleptic of higher potency
(E) anticholinergic medication

422. Which of the following drugs has shown the greatest efficacy in the treatment of obsessive-compulsive disorder?

(A) Alprazolam (Xanax)
(B) Clomipramine (Anafranil)
(C) Propranolol (Inderal)
(D) Phenobarbital
(E) Lithium

423. All the following drugs are commonly used to treat anxiety disorders EXCEPT

(A) phenobarbital
(B) alprazolam (Xanax)
(C) buspirone (BuSpar)
(D) imipramine (Tofranil)
(E) phenelzine (Nardil)

424. All the following drugs have some degree of cross-tolerance and cross-dependence with benzodiazepines EXCEPT

(A) alcohol
(B) narcotic analgesics
(C) barbiturates
(D) lithium
(E) chloral hydrate

425. In the treatment of depression, which of the following drugs is LEAST likely to lower the seizure threshold?

(A) Alprazolam (Xanax)
(B) Maprotiline (Ludiomil and others)
(C) Bupropion (Wellbutrin)
(D) Clomipramine (Anafranil)
(E) Amoxapine (Asendin)

426. All the following are capable of increasing plasma levels of lithium EXCEPT

(A) thiazide diuretics
(B) indomethacin
(C) fasting and low-salt diets
(D) phenylbutazone
(E) high intake of coffee

427. All the following statements about carbamazepine are true EXCEPT

(A) it is used in the treatment of mania
(B) it is used in the treatment of severe anxiety disorders
(C) it may cause fatal aplastic anemia
(D) it is potentially hepatotoxic
(E) it has mild anticholinergic activity

428. The anticholinergic syndrome may occur with overdoses of all the following drugs EXCEPT

(A) tricyclic antidepressants
(B) antipsychotics
(C) antihistamines
(D) antiparkinsonian agents
(E) anticholinesterase drugs

429. The anticholinergic syndrome may present with a mixture or predominance of either peripheral or central symptoms, including all the following EXCEPT

(A) delirium with disorientation
(B) agitation and restlessness
(C) marked sweating
(D) mydriasis
(E) increased body temperature

430. Which of the following drugs is a tricyclic antidepressant?

(A) Fluoxetine (Prozac)
(B) Nortriptyline (Pamelor, Aventyl)
(C) Phenelzine (Nardil)
(D) Tranylcypromine (Parnate)
(E) Clonazepam (Klonopin)

431. A 25-year-old woman gives a history of having used 30 mg/day of diazepam (Valium) for the past 20 months. Which of the following statements is most likely to be true?

(A) There is a small chance she is physically dependent
(B) She is almost certainly physically dependent
(C) She is probably not psychologically dependent
(D) She is probably not physically dependent, but is psychologically habituated
(E) Concern about physical dependency is not necessary at this dosage level

432. All the following drugs have been known to cause adverse interactions with monoamine oxidase inhibitors (MAOIs) EXCEPT

(A) chlorpromazine
(B) amphetamines and cocaine
(C) CoTylenol and Actifed
(D) clomipramine (Anafranil)
(E) meperidine (Demerol)

433. Side effects of the antipsychotic drugs include all the following EXCEPT

(A) priapism
(B) galactorrhea
(C) amenorrhea
(D) retrograde ejaculation
(E) increased appetite and weight gain

434. All the following statements about electroconvulsive therapy (ECT) are true EXCEPT

(A) the principal indication is for the treatment of severe depression
(B) it may be particularly effective in patients with delusional depression
(C) it may be of benefit in the treatment of manic excitement
(D) it is a procedure with a relatively high mortality
(E) it may be associated with impairment of memory

Items 435–436

A 29-year-old woman is brought into the hospital by her husband after having charged her credit card to the limit while buying 40 pairs of identical shoes. Her husband reports she has not slept in 2 days and paces the house all night. Her speech is pressured and its content difficult to follow. Two weeks earlier she had been extremely depressed. The diagnosis of bipolar disorder, manic, is made.

435. Before starting the patient on lithium, all the following tests should be done EXCEPT

(A) BUN and creatinine
(B) chest x-ray
(C) thyroid panel
(D) ECG
(E) pregnancy test

436. For long-term control, therapeutic lithium levels are

(A) 0.4 to 0.8 mg%
(B) 0.8 to 1.8 mg%
(C) 0.2 to 0.4 meq/L
(D) 0.6 to 1.2 meq/L
(E) 1 to 1.5 meq/g

437. Early central nervous system signs of lithium toxicity include all the following EXCEPT

(A) seizures
(B) ataxia
(C) tremor
(D) confusion
(E) dysarthria

438. Persons taking phenothiazine medication may develop tolerance to all the following effects of the drug EXCEPT

(A) sedation
(B) lightheadedness
(C) hypotension
(D) extrapyramidal reactions
(E) antipsychotic actions

439. All the following symptoms are commonly associated with a drug withdrawal syndrome involving central nervous system depressants EXCEPT

(A) lowered pulse, respiration, and body temperature
(B) tremor
(C) grand mal convulsions
(D) muscle aches
(E) gastrointestinal upset

440. All the following are true statements about fluoxetine (Prozac) EXCEPT

(A) the usual starting dosage is 20 mg/day
(B) its action is believed to be particularly on serotonergic neurons
(C) sedation is the most commonly encountered side effect
(D) it is commonly used to treat depression
(E) there has been speculation that it may show promise as an anti-obsessional drug

441. All the following statements about clozapine (Clozaril) are true EXCEPT

(A) it is a dibenzodiazepine drug
(B) it has a milligram equivalence to chlorpromazine of 2:1
(C) extrapyramidal side effects are common
(D) it may cause agranulocytosis
(E) it is associated with a risk for seizures

442. Propranolol (Inderal) is contraindicated in patients with

(A) hypertension
(B) asthma
(C) angina
(D) cardiac arrhythmias
(E) anxiety disorders

443. The half-life of a drug refers to

(A) how long the drug will last unused
(B) how long it takes to produce the drug
(C) how long the drug will remain at least one-half active
(D) how long it will take to metabolize one-half the drug
(E) the temperature a drug must be kept at to keep it from losing half its potency

444. A double-blind crossover drug study means

(A) the subject does not know whether he or she is getting drug or placebo during the study and is not told after completion of the study
(B) the researcher does not know if the subject is getting drug or placebo and is not told after completion of the study
(C) the subject is not told what he or she is taking and is switched from drug to placebo in mid-study
(D) neither the patient nor the researcher knows whether drug or placebo is being used, and a switch is made in mid-study
(E) none of the above

445. The benzodiazepine antianxiety drug with the fastest absorption from the gastrointestinal tract is

(A) alprazolam (Xanax)
(B) lorazepam (Ativan)
(C) prazepam (Centrex)
(D) diazepam (Valium)
(E) clorazepate (Tranxene)

446. Depression is a not uncommon side effect of

(A) insulin
(B) cortisone
(C) penicillin
(D) imipramine (Tofranil)
(E) bupropion (Wellbutrin)

447. Clozapine (Clozaril) is one of the newer drugs used to treat chronic and refractory

(A) obsessive-compulsive disorder
(B) dissociative disorder
(C) panic disorder
(D) Alzheimer's disease
(E) schizophrenia

448. All the following are symptoms commonly associated with tardive dyskinesia EXCEPT

(A) lip smacking or lip sucking
(B) tongue movements
(C) facial grimacing
(D) fine tremors of the upper extremities
(E) choreoathetoid movements of fingers and hands

449. A 60-year-old man who is taking lithium carbonate is admitted to a hospital because of cardiac disease. Even if his lithium dosage remained the same, all the following would be expected to increase his plasma lithium level EXCEPT

(A) associated renal disease
(B) thiazide diuretics
(C) ibuprofen (Motrin)
(D) low-sodium diet
(E) caffeine

450. Which of the following antipsychotics is the most potent?

(A) Chlorpromazine (Thorazine)
(B) Thiothixene (Navane)
(C) Trifluoperazine (Stelazine)
(D) Haloperidol (Haldol)
(E) Thioridazine (Mellaril)

451. All the following symptoms are associated with neuroleptic malignant syndrome EXCEPT

(A) hypothermia
(B) rigidity
(C) confusion
(D) autonomic dysfunction
(E) rhabdomyolysis

452. Side effects commonly associated with tricyclic antidepressants include all the following EXCEPT

(A) blurred vision
(B) diarrhea
(C) dry mouth
(D) urinary retention
(E) tachycardia

453. A 22-year-old man was being treated with fluoxetine (Prozac) for depression, while his twin brother was being treated for depression with an monoamine oxidase (MAO) inhibitor. Because of his increasing despair, the first man began to add his brother's MAO inhibitor to his daily fluoxetine. He soon began having visual hallucinations, became confused, and developed severe myoclonic jerks. On examination he was noted to be flushed and diaphoretic and to have a temperature of 39.44°C (103°F). The most likely diagnosis would be

(A) meningitis
(B) cerebral vascular incident
(C) neuroleptic malignant syndrome
(D) serotonin syndrome
(E) anticholinergic syndrome

454. A man who has agitated depression is started on the following medications (in daily doses): imipramine, 150 mg; perphenazine, 32 mg; and benztropine mesylate (Cogentin), 2 mg. One week later, his wife reports that he has been unusually forgetful during the last 4 days and that last night he awoke unusually confused about where he was. On physical examination, the man appears slightly flushed, his skin and palms are dry, and his heart rate is fast. He is slow to remember the date and has trouble concentrating. He showed none of these symptoms during his appointment last week. The diagnosis is

(A) anticholinergic syndrome
(B) neuroleptic syndrome
(C) schizophreniform psychosis
(D) toxic brain syndrome
(E) cerebrovascular accident

455. True statements about toxicity and dependence in the clinical use of benzodiazepines include all the following EXCEPT

(A) these agents are extremely lethal in overdose
(B) these agents are more lethal when combined with alcohol
(C) the potential for dependency is relatively low
(D) the potential for addiction is relatively low
(E) these agents must be used with caution with sedative drugs

456. The duration of action of a single dose of fluphenazine decanoate (Prolixin Decanoate) is

(A) 30 min
(B) 2 h
(C) 3 days
(D) 2 to 4 weeks
(E) 2 to 3 months

457. The minimum daily dosage of chlorpromazine (Thorazine) needed to produce a therapeutic effect in most psychotic persons is

(A) 10 mg
(B) 50 mg
(C) 300 mg
(D) 800 mg
(E) 1500 mg

458. The antimanic effect of lithium usually is observed within

(A) less than 24 h
(B) 1 to 4 days
(C) 5-14 days
(D) 30-40 days
(E) 2-3 months

459. The mechanism of action of antipsychotic drugs currently is believed to involve blockade at receptor sites for which of the following compounds?

(A) Histamine
(B) Dopamine
(C) Acetylcholine
(D) Epinephrine
(E) Gamma-aminobutyric acid

460. Which of the following drugs has the most pronounced anticholinergic effects?

(A) Amitriptyline
(B) Perphenazine
(C) Chlordiazepoxide
(D) Lithium
(E) Desipramine

461. Severe reactions and death have been reported in persons who had been taking an MAO inhibitor and then were given

(A) chlorpromazine
(B) diazepam
(C) lithium
(D) imipramine
(E) phenobarbital

462. Which of the following drugs is LEAST sedating?

(A) Chlorpromazine
(B) Imipramine
(C) Diazepam
(D) Lithium
(E) Haloperidol

463. In the treatment of persons in alcoholic withdrawal, chlordiazepoxide (Librium) commonly is used in daily doses as high as

(A) 20 mg
(B) 50 mg
(C) 400 mg
(D) 1000 mg
(E) 2000 mg

464. In the order presented, the medications thioridazine (Mellaril), chlorpromazine, perphenazine (Trilafon), and haloperidol (Haldol) are characterized by

(A) increasing hypotensive effects but decreasing sedative effects
(B) increasing hypotensive effects but decreasing extrapyramidal effects
(C) increasing extrapyramidal effects but decreasing anticholinergic effects
(D) increasing anticholinergic effects but decreasing hypotensive effects
(E) increasing sedative effects but decreasing anticholinergic effects

465. During a 2-month period, a 72-year-old woman who has senile dementia becomes increasingly withdrawn, shows little interest in food, has trouble sleeping, and appears to become more severely demented. Her medical status is unchanged. Which of the following courses of treatment would be the most reasonable?

(A) Bedtime sedation to improve sleep
(B) Diazepam, 5 mg three times daily
(C) A trial of tricyclic antidepressants
(D) A trial of perphenazine, 4 mg three times daily
(E) None of the above, because her condition is untreatable

466. The serum level of lithium at which therapeutic benefit levels off and side effects increase usually is considered to be

(A) 0.5 meq/L
(B) 1.0 meq/L
(C) 1.5 meq/L
(D) 2.0 meq/L
(E) 3.0 meq/L

467. Clinical response to an adequate dosage of tricyclic antidepressants typically occurs how long after initiation of treatment?

(A) 1 to 2 h
(B) 4 to 8 h
(C) 12 to 24 h
(D) 3 to 10 days
(E) 21 to 30 days

468. Physicians caring for persons who have taken an overdose of tricyclic antidepressants should pay special attention to which of the following clinical indicators?

(A) Renal output
(B) Cardiac rhythm
(C) Serum levels of bilirubin
(D) Bowel sounds
(E) Serum levels of glutamic oxaloacetic transaminase (SGOT)

469. The usual daily dosage range of imipramine that is effective for the treatment of most depressed adults is

(A) 2 to 25 mg
(B) 25 to 50 mg
(C) 75 to 125 mg
(D) 150 to 300 mg
(E) 200 to 800 mg

470. Tricyclic antidepressants block the action of which of the following drugs?

(A) Chlorpromazine
(B) Guanethidine (Ismelin)
(C) Diazepam (Valium)
(D) Phenytoin (Dilantin)
(E) Quinidine

471. Gilles de la Tourette's syndrome is a childhood disorder that often begins with facial tics and progresses to multiple tics, grimacing, and spasmodic utterances. Patients with this disease are usually treated with

(A) chlordiazepoxide
(B) haloperidol
(C) methylphenidate (Ritalin)
(D) tranylcypromine (Parnate)
(E) protriptyline (Vivactil)

472. In elderly persons, increased confusion and paradoxical agitation are most likely to be associated with administration of which of the following sleep-inducing medications?

(A) Secobarbital (Seconal)
(B) Flurazepam (Dalmane)
(C) Chloral hydrate
(D) Chlorpromazine
(E) Amitriptyline

473. Epinephrine is contraindicated for the treatment of hypotension in persons taking

(A) diazepam
(B) lithium
(C) amitriptyline
(D) imipramine
(E) chlorpromazine

474. A chronically depressed patient seriously overdoses with a tricyclic antidepressant. All the following signs and symptoms are likely to be seen EXCEPT

(A) hypotension
(B) cardiac arrhythmia
(C) seizure activity
(D) delirium
(E) serenity and indifference

475. A patient reports that she has become depressed with the onset of winter every year for the past 6 years. A diagnosis of major depressive disorder with seasonal pattern is made. It is likely that the patient would have a trial of treatment with

(A) phototherapy
(B) biofeedback
(C) electroconvulsive therapy
(D) benzodiazepines
(E) steroid medication

DIRECTIONS: The group of questions below consists of lettered options followed by numbered items. For each numbered item, select the appropriate lettered option(s). Each lettered option may be used once, more than once, or not at all. **Choose exactly the number of options indicated following each item.**

Items 476–479

For each patient with side effects due to treatment with high-potency neuroleptic medication, select the most likely diagnosis.

(A) Parkinsonism
(B) Akathisia
(C) Neuroleptic malignant syndrome
(D) Dystonia
(E) Anticholinergic syndrome
(F) Seizure activity
(G) Rabbit syndrome
(H) Tremor
(I) Akinesia

476. A 19-year-old phencyclidine abuser is hospitalized, and 7 days after the initiation of haloperidol is noted to be pacing and jiggling his legs. **(SELECT 1 DIAGNOSIS)**

477. A 35-year-old woman with a diagnosis of chronic schizophrenia is hospitalized with a recurrent episode of acute psychosis. She is extremely agitated and combative and is placed on high doses of a high-potency neuroleptic. Shortly after initiation of treatment, she becomes mute and delirious and develops a high temperature, muscle rigidity, an increase in the level of muscle enzymes, and leukocytosis. **(SELECT 1 DIAGNOSIS)**

478. An adolescent with mental retardation is admitted with a first-time psychotic reaction of unknown etiology. Two days after the initiation of neuroleptic medication, he begins screaming that something is wrong with his eyes. On examination they appear to be rolled upward and frozen in that position. **(SELECT 1 DIAGNOSIS)**

479. A 55-year-old man has a 30-year history of schizophrenia, and because of agitation and paranoid behavior, he has been on neuroleptic medication quite steadily for many years. He lives in a board-and-care facility, the staff of which noted that he has lately developed a stiff gait, a pill-rolling type of tremor, and a rather expressionless face. **(SELECT 1 DIAGNOSIS)**

Psychopharmacology and Other Therapies

Answers

420. The answer is E. *(Kaplan, 6/e, pp 988–994.)* Schizophrenia is a chronic psychotic disorder. It is responsive to diverse psychopharmacologic treatments. The mainstay of treatment for schizophrenia is the group of medications called antipsychotics, or neuroleptics. They include the phenothiazines (Thorazine, Mellaril, Stelazine, Prolixin), butyrophenones (Haldol), thioxanthenes (Navane), and others. Risperidone and olanzapine are newer drugs that have been introduced as a first line of treatment. While lithium has been used successfully to augment antipsychotic medications, it is not a primary treatment for the psychotic symptoms of schizophrenia.

421. The answer is B. *(Kaplan, 6/e, p 995.)* Akathisia has not been found to be responsive to the anticholinergic medications used to treat parkinsonism. Benzodiazepines and diphenhydramine (Benadryl) have shown limited usefulness. The medication most commonly used is propranolol in relatively small dosage.

422. The answer is B. *(Schatzberg, p 150.)* Clomipramine is a tricyclic drug, and its chemical structure resembles that of imipramine. It appears to have an anti-obsessional effect that is not as readily apparent with other antidepressant drugs. Clomipramine has been studied in both children and adults, and its efficacy is thought to be related to effects on the serotonin system.

423. The answer is A. *(Hales, 2/e, pp 944–962.)* Phenobarbital was historically used to treat anxiety, but is rarely used today. There are other, more effective antianxiety agents, such as alprazolam. Also, the barbiturates have a considerable potential for addiction and problems of withdrawal. Antidepressants such as tricyclics and monoamine oxidase inhibitors are often used to treat panic disorder, and buspirone is a newer agent used to treat chronic anxiety states.

424. The answer is D. *(Hales, 2/e, p 960.)* The long-term use of benzodiazepines results in tolerance to both the hypnotic and anxiolytic effects, and this is what leads many patients to increase either their dose or frequency. Cross-tolerance develops to other CNS depressants such as alcohol, barbiturates, narcotic analgesics, chloral hydrate, and other sedative hypnotics.

Cocaine abusers may use benzodiazepines to counteract the stimulant effects of that drug, but there is no cross-tolerance between these two drugs.

425. The answer is A. *(Hales, 2/e, p 938.)* All antidepressants appear to lower seizure threshold, though this is mostly a clinical problem in patients with preexisting seizure disorder, those withdrawing from alcohol or sedatives, and those with eating disorders. With tricyclic antidepressants the risk is probably less than 1 percent, although with clomipramine and amoxapine the risk may be somewhat greater. Both maprotiline and bupropion have been associated with seizure activity, especially at higher dose ranges. There is some clinical use of alprazolam as an antidepressant, and benzodiazepines raise rather than lower seizure threshold.

426. The answer is E. *(Kaplan, 6/e, pp 2029–2030.)* When a patient is stabilized on lithium, and a thiazide diuretic is added in ignorance, the lithium level can double or reach toxicity. Low-salt diets and fasting can also decrease excretion of lithium, thereby increasing plasma levels. Indomethacin and phenylbutazone (nonsteroidal anti-inflammatory agents) have been reported to significantly decrease excretion of lithium. Clinicians should be alert to the possibility of a high intake of coffee interfering with achieving therapeutic levels of lithium.

427. The answer is B. *(Schatzberg, pp 351–359.)* Carbamazepine has been found to be effective in the treatment of acute manic episodes, as well as in the prophylactic treatment of mania. It is not used in the treatment of anxiety disorders. One problem with the use of this drug relates to its potential for hepatotoxicity and hematologic toxicity, including aplastic anemia. Since the drug has mild anticholinergic activity, some patients may complain of blurred vision, constipation, and dry mouth. Other complaints include dizziness, ataxia, and drowsiness.

428. The answer is E. *(Kaplan, 6/e, pp 1163, 1921–1923.)* Many drugs used with psychiatric patients have both peripheral and central anticholinergic effects. Most notably included are the tricyclic and some other antidepressants, as well as antipsychotics, antiparkinsonian agents, some hypnotic drugs, and antihistamines. Either overdose or combinations of these drugs may produce sufficient anticholinergic effects to result in an anticholinergic crisis. Anticholinesterase drugs, such as physostigmine or pyridostigmine, are used to treat this syndrome.

429. The answer is C. *(Kaplan, 6/e, p 1922.)* The anticholinergic syndrome may be associated with delirium and confusion, delusions, and hallucinations. The patient is typically agitated and anxious, shows motor restlessness, and may have myoclonic jerks and choreoathetoid movements. The peripheral syndrome may present constipation and decreased bowel sounds, increased pupillary size, urinary retention, motor incoordination, and increased body temperature. The anticholinergic activity produces anhidrosis rather than sweating.

430. The answer is B. *(Schatzberg, pp 141–154.)* Tricyclic drugs in common use include imipramine, desipramine, and nortriptyline. They are usually employed in the treatment of panic disorder and depression. While similar in their antidepressant and antianxiety effects, they are associated with different side-effect profiles. For example, desipramine has less anticholinergic effect than imipramine, and nortriptyline is less likely to cause orthostatic hypotension.

431. The answer is B. *(Schuckit, 4/e, pp 28–32.)* The benzodiazepines are best used for short-term treatment (2 to 4 weeks). They are not effective over a long period of time, and one can expect a rebound increase in symptoms if the drugs are stopped. Benzodiazepines, especially diazepam, are very common drugs of abuse. The development of physical dependence relates to the drug dose and the length of time it is taken. Physical withdrawal has been reported with diazepam in the clinical dose range of 10 to 20 mg/day when taken over a period of weeks to months. This woman is probably physically dependent, and a drug withdrawal syndrome must be considered. Psychological dependency accompanies physical dependency.

432. The answer is A. *(Hales, 2/e, pp 939–943.)* A number of medications and drugs can cause severe reactions in patients being treated with MAOIs. Hypertensive crisis can occur when a patient is switched abruptly from one MAOI to another or with the ingestion of food or beverage with a high tyramine content. This may also occur with stimulant drugs or with sympathomimetics such as those found in many over-the-counter preparations that contain phenylpropanolamine, pseudoephedrine, or phenylephrine. Hyperpyrexia, hyperreflexia, muscle rigidity, seizures, hypotension, and death have occurred with meperidine (Demerol). Some antidepressants, notably clomipramine (Anafranil) and possibly fluoxetine (Prozac), have caused death.

433. The answer is A. *(Hales, 2/e, pp 900–922.)* Antipsychotic drugs have a number of hormonal, sexual, and hypothalamic side effects. They increase prolactin release from the anterior pituitary, which causes galactorrhea, decreased menstruation, and diminished libido. Circulating levels of testosterone are also decreased, which may contribute to the decreased libido observed in some males. Both sexes may complain of delayed, altered, or inadequate orgasms, including retrograde ejaculation, which is particularly noted with thioridazine (Mellaril). Appetite increase with weight gain can sometimes be marked and may be more common with the low-potency drugs. Priapism is not encountered with antipsychotic drugs but is occasionally associated with the antidepressant drug trazodone (Desyrel).

434. The answer is D. *(Hales, 2/e, pp 982–984.)* In general, ECT is a relatively safe procedure. The morbidity and mortality are not significantly greater than for general anesthesia. The mortality is approximately one per 10,000 patients. Its principal indication is in the treatment of severe depression, particularly delusional depression and depression unresponsive to antidepressant medication. It is also used in elderly patients who cannot tolerate the side effects of antipsychotic or antidepressant agents. ECT has been found useful in the treatment of acute manic excitement that cannot be otherwise controlled. Impairment of memory is a common but variable complaint of patients receiving this treatment.

435–436. The answers are 435-B, 436-D. *(Hales, 2/e, pp 962–971.)* Lithium is the drug of choice for bipolar disorders. Its advantages over neuroleptics include a greater degree of specificity and ease in monitoring plasma levels, and it does not produce tardive dyskinesia. Therapeutic blood levels for long-term maintenance are from 0.6 to 1.2 meq/L, and it has a serum half-life of about 24 h. Being a salt, it "competes" in the body with sodium and has effects on the heart, kidney, and thyroid. It can also cause birth defects. Unless indicated for another reason, a chest x-ray is not mandatory as a preadministration screen. Initial dosage is variable, but a test dose of 600 mg is often chosen to establish the regimen. The average adult usually requires 900 to 1200 mg/day for long-term control, and about 1800 mg/day for the treatment of acute mania.

437. The answer is A. *(Hales, 2/e, pp 969–970.)* Early signs of lithium toxicity include confusion, lethargy, coarse tremor, dysarthria, vomiting, diarrhea, and ataxia. When these signs occur, it is necessary to immediately discontinue lithium so as to allow the plasma level to decrease. If lithium is continued, hyperreflexia, muscle tremor and fasciculation, seizures, coma, and even death may result.

438. The answer is E. *(Hales, 2/e, pp 900–919.)* Most people develop tolerance to sedation and accommodate to the lightheadedness associated with the hypotensive side effects of phenothiazines. Antiparkinsonian drugs can sometimes be discontinued after 2 or 3 months because of tolerance to the extrapyramidal side effects. It is the fact that patients do not develop tolerance to the antipsychotic action of these drugs that allows them to be used for years, often at the same dosage, in maintenance therapy.

439. The answer is A. *(Schuckit, 4/e, pp 40–43.)* The drug withdrawal syndrome related to central nervous system depressants has a mixture of both physical and psychological symptoms. Patients often complain of gastrointestinal upset, muscle aches, and sometimes headache and malaise. The most common autonomic nervous system reaction would be increased pulse and respiration rates, labile blood pressure, and fever. Barbiturate withdrawal is associated with the danger of grand mal convulsions.

440. The answer is C. *(Schuckit, 4/e, pp 228–231.)* Fluoxetine (Prozac) was one of the most commonly prescribed antidepressants in the United States in 1990. Because of its effects on the serotonergic system, some clinicians have reported that it may have an anti-obsessional effect similar to that of clomipramine. The most common side effects of this drug relate to nervousness and difficulty sleeping. The usual starting dose is 20 mg/day, and this is a sufficient treatment level for many patients.

441. The answer is C. *(Hales, 2/e, pp 919–921.)* Clozapine is a dibenzodiazepine compound that has been demonstrated to be an effective antipsychotic, and it is most often used in the treatment of chronic schizophrenia. It has a 2:1 approximate potency when compared with chlorpromazine and has rare, if any, extrapyramidal side effects. Lowered seizure threshold and the potential for agranulocytosis are two of the major concerns in prescribing this drug.

442. The answer is B. *(Kaplan, 6/e, pp 253, 1243, 1915–1919.)* Propranolol acts to block beta-noradrenergic receptors in the peripheral sympathetic nervous system and probably also acts centrally. It blocks both cardiac and pulmonary beta-receptors; the latter are responsible for bronchial dilation, and thus propranolol is contraindicated in asthma. It is also to be avoided or used with great caution in patients with diabetes because of its considerable effects on fat and sugar metabolism. The drug is used to block the peripheral symptoms of anxiety, such as tachycardia and tremor, and is also used to lower blood pressure, to prevent angina pectoris, and to control certain cardiac arrhythmias.

443. The answer is D. *(Kaplan, 6/e, pp 1895–1898.)* The half-life of a drug refers to how long it will take the body to metabolize one-half of the drug. Knowing the half-life is important in determining how often a drug should be administered. It is also helpful to know where a drug is metabolized. For example, drugs excreted via the renal system will be affected by any form of altered renal function. Organ pathology can greatly alter the normal half-life of a medication.

444. The answer is D. *(Kaplan, 6/e, pp 1936, 2782.)* Double-blind crossover studies are done to control for individual differences in drug response and the placebo effect. They are conducted with neither the subject (patient) nor the researcher (physician) knowing whether the substance being taken is placebo or drug. This is double-blind. Crossover refers to changing from drug to placebo, or vice versa, in mid-study, again without knowledge of the subject or researcher.

445. The answer is D. *(Kaplan, 6/e, pp 1934–1936.)* The rapidity of onset of a benzodiazepine drug is largely determined by the rate at which it is absorbed from the intestinal tract. Diazepam is absorbed rapidly and produces prompt effects following a single oral dose. The peak concentration of diazepam may occur within an hour. The other listed drugs are absorbed more slowly. Clorazepate is the next fastest, followed by alprazolam and lorazepam, and prazepam is the slowest.

446. The answer is B. *(Kaplan, 6/e, p 1597.)* A number of drugs are not uncommonly associated with the side effect of depression. These include the adrenocortical steroids, such as prednisone and cortisone; estrogens and progestins found in birth control pills; and thyroid medications. Such drugs may cause depression directly or upon withdrawal. Penicillin is not associated with depression, and both imipramine and bupropion are used to treat depression.

447. The answer is E. *(Kaplan, 6/e, pp 919–921.)* Clozapine (Clozaril) is a relatively new drug used to treat chronic and refractory schizophrenia. A significant number of patients using this drug have developed a potentially fatal agranulocytosis. For this reason it is generally not employed until it is established that the patient is unresponsive to the normally prescribed neuroleptics. A special system has been established to monitor patients on this drug.

448. The answer is D. *(Kaplan, 6/e, p 912.)* Tardive dyskinesia consists of abnormal involuntary movements. It is seen in some patients who have received long-term antipsychotic medication. Chewing motions, lip smacking or sucking, and tongue movements are common. The patient may demonstrate facial grimacing, and choreoathetoid movements of the fingers and hands are also seen and on occasion can extend to the trunk and extremities.

449. The answer is E. *(Hales, 2/e, pp 965–971.)* Lithium carbonate is eliminated from the body by urinary excretion. Both low-sodium diets and thiazide diuretics increase plasma lithium concentration by increasing reabsorption of lithium by the kidney. Ibuprofen is associated with increased levels of lithium, while caffeine and other xanthines cause decreased blood levels by increasing the excretion of lithium. Patients receiving these and other drugs that affect lithium excretion must have frequent monitoring of their lithium blood level.

450. The answer is D. *(Hales, 2/e, pp 900–919.)* The potency of an antipsychotic relates to its ability to block postsynaptic dopamine receptors. In general, the more potent the drug, the less sedating it is. Haloperidol is a high-potency neuroleptic, many times more potent than thioridazine, trifluoperazine, thiothixene, and chlorpromazine.

451. The answer is A. *(Schatzberg, p 629.)* The neuroleptic malignant syndrome is associated with administration of antipsychotic drugs. It characteristically is manifested by fever, not hypothermia. It is also associated with confusion, rigidity, and autonomic dysfunction. Normally the condition resolves with discontinuance of the antipsychotic drug, but the mortality may be as high as 20 percent.

452. The answer is B. *(Kaplan, 6/e, pp 2107–2108.)* Tricyclic antidepressants have anticholinergic properties. As a result they typically cause blurred vision, dry mouth, dizziness, tachycardia, and palpitations. They generally cause constipation rather than diarrhea. More serious side effects include urinary retention and paralytic ileus.

453. The answer is D. *(Hales, 2/e, p 939.)* Excessive stimulation of the serotoninergic system can result in the serotonin syndrome. It most commonly occurs in patients treated with two serotoninergic drugs, such as an SSRI and an MAO inhibitor. The usual symptoms include lethargy, restlessness, confusion, flushing, diaphoresis, tremor, and myoclonic jerks. Hyperthermia, myoclonus, and rigor may develop. Medication must be discontinued immediately, and emergency medical treatment undertaken because the condition has the potential to progress to rhabdomyolysis, acidosis, respiratory compromise, and renal failure secondary to myoglobinuria.

454. The answer is D. *(Kaplan, 6/e, pp 1922–1923.)* Phenothiazines, tricyclic antidepressants, and antiparkinsonian agents (such as benztropine mesylate) all have anticholinergic properties. The action of these drugs becomes additive when they are administered in combination. It is not uncommon for persons receiving such a combination to show evidence of a mild organic brain syndrome, including difficulty in concentrating, impaired short-term memory, and disorientation, which often is more noticeable at night. Dry skin and palms are especially suggestive of atropinism.

455. The answer is A. *(Hales, 2/e, pp 377–378, 517–518.)* While clinicians were initially quite concerned about the potential for addiction and dependency with benzodiazepines, experience has shown that this is a relatively low-risk though significant potential problem. Death from overdose is not common, except when these agents are taken in combination with other drugs, especially sedatives and alcohol. It is believed that alcoholics have a greater likelihood of becoming dependent on these drugs.

456. The answer is D. *(Hales, 2/e, pp 444, 9021. Schatzberg, p 620.)* Fluphenazine decanoate is the decanoic-acid ester of fluphenazine (Prolixin). Esterification of fluphenazine slows its release from the injection site. The usual duration of action of intramuscular fluphenazine decanoate averages 2 to 4 weeks with maintenance treatment. Dosage must be individualized.

457. The answer is C. *(Kaplan, 6/e, p 990.)* A number of controlled studies have demonstrated that chlorpromazine (Thorazine), when given in daily doses of 300 mg or greater, was a significantly more effective antipsychotic agent than was placebo. At doses below 300 mg, this effect was not demonstrated clearly, although other effects of chlorpromazine are noted at lower dosages.

458. The answer is C. *(Kaplan, 6/e, pp 1169–1170, 2030.)* The antimanic effect of lithium on manic patients usually is observed in 5 to 14 days. If a patient is agitated, sleepless, or otherwise unmanageable during the initiation of lithium therapy, an antipsychotic agent (either haloperidol or a phenothiazine) may be used.

459. The answer is B. *(Kaplan, 6/e, pp 1994–1997.)* Antipsychotic drugs block dopamine receptor sites. Blockade of dopamine receptors in the limbic system is believed to be responsible for the antipsychotic effects. Blockade in the basal ganglia results in the "extrapyramidal" side effects of the drugs.

460. The answer is A. *(Kaplan, 6/e, p 1163.)* The anticholinergic or atropinic side effects of the tricyclic antidepressants can be pronounced. Dry mouth, for example, is routinely produced by therapeutic dosages of tricyclic antidepressant agents. Among the tricyclic antidepressants, amitriptyline is one of the most potent anticholinergic agents and desipramine the least. The anticholinergic effects of the phenothiazines are less strong. Lithium and the benzodiazepines are not atropinic.

461. The answer is D. *(Kaplan, 6/e, p 1163.)* Severe reactions, even death, have been reported in persons receiving an MAO inhibitor who were given a high dose of tricyclic antidepressant. This observation has led to the belief that the two drugs might be a lethal combination. A waiting period of a week or more is indicated when switching from an MAO inhibitor to a tricyclic antidepressant.

462. The answer is D. *(Kaplan, 6/e, pp 1171–1172.)* Lithium is one of the few major drugs used in psychiatry that does not commonly produce some sedation or euphoria in normal subjects. This observation appears to be related to the clinical finding that persons receiving lithium therapy, unlike those taking phenothiazines or tricyclic antidepressants, seldom complain of feeling drugged.

463. The answer is C. *(Schuckit, 4/e, pp 105–107.)* Chlordiazepoxide (Librium) frequently is used in the treatment of persons in alcoholic withdrawal. Dosage must be sufficient to relieve tremors and agitation. Doses will vary, but commonly will be in the range of 200 to 400 mg/day.

464. The answer is C. *(Kaplan, 6/e, p 2008.)* The antipsychotic drugs listed in the question are arranged in order of increasing extrapyramidal effects and decreasing anticholinergic, hypotensive, and sedative effects. Knowledge of the position of a drug along this side-effect gradient is useful in selecting the most suitable drug for a given individual. It should be remembered, too, that individuals experience a variety of side effects for which they exhibit variable tolerances.

465. The answer is C. *(DSM-IV, p 344.)* Depression in elderly persons, especially those who already have some evidence of dementia, may suggest deterioration of the organic process. The differentiation of progressing dementia from depression may be impossible. If the onset of symptoms is reasonably abrupt (1 or 2 months) and the patient has other signs suggestive of depression (e.g., changes in sleeping and eating habits) accompanied by motor retardation or agitation, depression should be considered. It certainly is preferable to consider a trial of antidepressants, which might be beneficial, rather than to assume a person's dementia is progressive and untreatable.

Potential worsening of this condition, because of the side effects of medication, is a problem.

466. The answer is C. *(Kaplan, 6/e, pp 2023–2024.)* The therapeutic serum concentration of lithium for manic patients is 0.6 to 1.2 meq/L. In maintenance therapy, a level of 0.6 to 1.0 meq/L usually is sufficient. At lithium levels higher than 1.5 meq/L, the incidence of side effects rapidly increases.

467. The answer is D. *(Kaplan, 6/e, p 1164.)* Improvement in the condition of a depressed patient receiving a tricyclic antidepressant at an adequate dosage often appears in 3 to 10 days, is usually present by 2 weeks, but sometimes may not occur until the third week. For this reason, many clinicians feel that an adequate trial of a tricyclic antidepressant requires at least 3 weeks of treatment. Although patients who have a partial response may continue to improve, those who have not responded to treatment at the end of 3 weeks either require treatment at higher dosage or need different treatment.

468. The answer is B. *(Kaplan, 6/e, p 2109.)* Cardiac arrhythmia, which sometimes can be fatal, is the most common dangerous consequence of an overdose of tricyclic antidepressant. For this reason, electrocardiographic monitoring is advised for persons who have taken a significant overdose. Physostigmine can be used to reverse the anticholinergic effects.

469. The answer is D. *(Kaplan, 6/e, p 2100.)* The effective dosage range of imipramine for most patients is 75 to 250 mg daily. In a few persons, dosages above or below this range may be required because of unusual pharmacokinetics. A common error is to continue treatment at inadequate dosage levels.

470. The answer is B. *(Schatzberg, p 786.)* Guanethidine (Ismelin) produces its antihypertensive effect after its uptake by peripheral noradrenergic neurons. Because tricyclic antidepressants block this uptake mechanism, guanethidine cannot reach its site of action.

471. The answer is B. *(Kaplan, 6/e, pp 2334–2335.)* Haloperidol has been reported to reduce symptoms by 90 percent in most people who have Gilles de la Tourette's syndrome. The dosage prescribed by clinicians ranges considerably. Ritalin is sometimes used to treat tic disorders.

472. The answer is A. *(Kaplan, 6/e, p 2606.)* Although any sedating drug has the potential for adding to the confusion of an elderly person, the barbiturates are most frequently associated with paradoxical agitation or excitement. Chloral hydrate and flurazepam (Dalmane) are useful in treating insomnia in older persons. In the treatment of insomnia in an elderly patient who has either psychosis or depression, an antipsychotic or antidepressant drug may be indicated.

473. The answer is E. *(Kaplan, 6/e, p 996.)* Chlorpromazine, through its alpha-adrenergic blockade, blocks the alpha-stimulating effect of epinephrine and allows the beta-stimulating effect to predominate. Thus, instead of having a pressor effect, epinephrine produces hypotension. Hypotension in a person receiving chlorpromazine should be treated with volume expansion and administration of norepinephrine, which has alpha-stimulating but not beta-stimulating effects.

474. The answer is E. *(Hales, 2/e, p 939.)* Overdose with a tricyclic antidepressant (TCA) is a serious emergency, with a significant risk of cardiac death. Typically one encounters hypotension (though hypertension may be seen in serious overdose), cardiac abnormalities, agitation or delirium, and sometimes seizure activity. TCA overdose requires immediate medical management.

475. The answer is A. *(Kaplan, 6/e, p 2145.)* Seasonal depression, which is associated with decreased daylight hours, typically occurs at the onset of winter and fades in the spring. It often has the symptoms of an atypical depression with weight gain and hypersomnia. It is commonly treated with the MAO inhibitor antidepressant drugs or the SSRIs. The phototherapy of exposure to very bright light of 2500 lux or more is believed to be effective. Benzodiazepines, biofeedback, and steroid medication are not employed to treat major depressive symptoms. Electroconvulsive therapy would not commonly be considered for such a patient.

476–479. The answers are 476-B, 477-C, 478-D, 479-A. *(Kaplan, 6/e, pp 662–664, 994–996.)* Antipsychotic medication, and particularly the high-potency neuroleptic medications, are associated with a number of potential side effects. Akathisia is a common one and is sometimes referred to as the "restless legs syndrome." Typically these patients pace and jiggle their legs frequently in an attempt to relieve the troublesome feelings.

The neuroleptic malignant syndrome is a serious and potentially lethal condition that can occur at any time during treatment with antipsychotic medication. The incidence is believed to be approximately 0.1 to 1 percent. The syndrome is sometimes mistakenly interpreted as catatonia because of the muscle rigidity.

Acute dystonic reactions are sometimes seen in patients treated with neuroleptic medication, usually in the early stages and most often in those not previously treated with these medications. There is characteristic muscle spasm in discrete groups, often the neck or eye musculature, resulting in torticollis or oculogyric crisis. The latter is characterized by a forced upward gaze.

Parkinsonism is a complication that may be seen in psychiatric patients taking antipsychotic medication. There is usually akinesis, a stiff gait with diminished arm swing, and sometimes pill-rolling tremor. Cogwheel rigidity is noted on examination, and often the patient's face and speech seem expressionless and monotonous.

Law and Ethics in Psychiatry

DIRECTIONS: Each item below contains a question or incomplete statement followed by suggested responses. Select the **one best** response to each question.

480. A 50-year-old man is suing his psychiatrist for malpractice. This resulted from his having developed an acute serotonin syndrome while under treatment for depression. For a successful lawsuit, the former patient must prove that all the following elements of malpractice are present EXCEPT

(A) negligence
(B) duty
(C) direct causation
(D) intent
(E) damage

481. When a subpoena is delivered ordering release of psychiatric records, the psychiatrist

(A) must release the records immediately
(B) may update and modify the records before releasing them
(C) may demand a judicial hearing before releasing them
(D) may release them only with the patient's permission
(E) may refuse to release them because of doctor-patient privilege

482. In the Cruzan case (Cruzan v. Director, 1990), the Supreme Court found that

(A) the mentally ill must have a guardian appointed to protect their rights
(B) mental illness is an appropriate defense for murder
(C) durable powers of attorney expire upon death
(D) alcoholic intoxication is not an appropriate defense to a charge of manslaughter
(E) a competent person has the right to refuse unwanted medical treatment

483. The standard for criminal responsibility in most U.S. federal courts is the

(A) product rule
(B) M'Naghten rule
(C) American Law Institute test
(D) irresistible impulse rule
(E) Currens test

484. Privileged communication means

(A) that psychiatrists have the privilege of disclosing information about a patient to other psychiatrists or physicians
(B) that the information revealed by psychiatrists at a probate hearing is handled as privileged
(C) that psychiatrists are granted by the court the "privilege" to disclose information about a specific patient
(D) that patients have the statutory right to prevent psychiatrists from disclosing confidential information
(E) none of the above

485. The landmark decision in Tarasoff v. Regents of California held that a therapist has an obligation to

(A) protect the confidentiality of information obtained during therapy
(B) warn the university when students are involved in any illegal activities
(C) report to university authorities the presence of a student who is involved in illegal drug sales
(D) warn the potential victim of a potentially violent patient
(E) give informed consent to patients of the student health center who are given neuroleptic medications

Items 486–487

A psychiatrist is called in to evaluate a wealthy 85-year-old man who is drawing up a new "last will" and is concerned that it might be challenged after his death on the basis of possible reduced mental capacity.

486. The psychiatric evaluation would be for the purpose of determining the patient's

(A) sanity versus insanity
(B) testamentary capacity
(C) ability to distinguish right from wrong
(D) judgmental capacity
(E) insight

487. The essential components of a valid will include all the following EXCEPT

(A) the absence of any axis I diagnosis
(B) knowledge of the nature and extent of one's assets
(C) knowledge of relatives and natural heirs
(D) knowledge that a will is being made
(E) freedom from undue influence

488. The most common cause of malpractice claims is

(A) drug overdose or addiction
(B) suicide
(C) improper sexual involvement
(D) failure to treat psychosis
(E) restraints

489. A patient with a family history of Huntington's disease wishes to select his nephew as the person to make decisions about health care if he should become incompetent. The necessary document is called a

(A) last testament
(B) durable power of attorney
(C) informed consent
(D) competency document
(E) contract

490. A patient is constantly critical of the psychiatrist and the psychiatric treatment. The physician is not legally bound to continue treatment if

(A) dismissed by the patient, who is believed to be competent
(B) the patient is given ample medication to last until a new therapist can be found
(C) the psychiatrist recommends the patient seek a new therapist
(D) the patient is uncooperative with the treatment
(E) the doctor explains the action to the family

491. A psychiatrist elicits a patient's cooperation in trying a new and experimental treatment. This is an example of informed consent, which involves providing information regarding all the following EXCEPT the

(A) nature of the procedure or treatment
(B) risks that are material, substantial, probable, or significant
(C) anticipated benefits and probability of success
(D) alternatives to this new treatment
(E) identity of recipients of a placebo versus the investigational medication

492. In Tarasoff-II, the second decision by the California Supreme Court, the original Tarasoff ruling was revised by

(A) requiring the warning of only "identifiable" potential victims
(B) imposing legal liabilty on police
(C) requiring hospitalization of patients deemed dangerous
(D) finding a duty to protect potential victims, not just warn them
(E) requiring use of neuroleptic medication

493. A male psychiatrist and his patient fall in love. The psychiatrist terminates treatment, and they begin a sexual relationship. All the following statements about the relevant moral and legal issues for the psychiatrist are true EXCEPT

(A) he is in violation of the American Psychiatric Association's guidelines for ethical conduct
(B) he is liable to malpractice suits, even if the patient consents
(C) he is in jeopardy of having his licence revoked
(D) he is not in legal or ethical jeopardy if he has allowed at least 3 months to elapse before beginning the sexual relationship
(E) he is liable for prosecution for rape

494. All the following are exceptions to the legal and ethical issue of *privilege* EXCEPT

(A) a court order exists
(B) the psychiatrist has not had contact with the patient for over 5 years
(C) the psychiatrist is the subject of a lawsuit by the patient
(D) the patient makes his or her mental state or condition a legal issue, such as emotional damage due to injury
(E) child-custody is the issue (some jurisdictions)

DIRECTIONS: The group of questions below consists of lettered options followed by numbered items. For each numbered item, select the appropriate lettered option(s). Each lettered option may be used once, more than once, or not at all. **Choose exactly the number of options indicated following each item.**

Items 495–500

Match each statement to the appropriate legal concept.

(A) M'Naghten rule
(B) Irresistible impulse rule
(C) American Law Institute: Model Penal Code
(D) Durham rule
(E) Mens rea elements

495. Psychiatric testimony should be addressed only to the issue of state of mind and criminal intent at the time of the crime. **(SELECT 1 CONCEPT)**

496. An insanity defense is the inability to know the nature and quality of the act being done or to know that what was being done was wrong. **(SELECT 1 CONCEPT)**

497. An accused is not criminally responsible if the unlawful act was the product of mental disease or mental defect. **(SELECT 1 CONCEPT)**

498. Criminal responsibility should not be excluded on the basis of those conditions that may have associated sociopathic behaviors, such as some personality disorders. **(SELECT 1 CONCEPT)**

499. "A person is not responsible for criminal conduct if at the time of such conduct as a result of mental disease or defect he lacks substantial capacity either to appreciate the criminality (wrongfulness) of his conduct or to conform his conduct to the requirements of the law." **(SELECT 1 CONCEPT)**

500. The defendant must have the volition (freedom of will) to refrain from the criminal act

Law and Ethics in Psychiatry

Answers

480. The answer is D. *(Kaplan, 6/e, pp 2748–2749.)* In a malpractice lawsuit, the plaintiff must show that the four elements of malpractice are present by a preponderance of evidence. These are the so-called four D's of malpractice: dereliction (negligence), duty, direct causation, and damages. The first means that the physician neglected to do something that is ordinarily a part of standard care, and this was a breach of duty of proper care owed by physicians to their patients. This must then have resulted in direct causation of the damages allegedly caused by the negligence.

481. The answer is C. *(Kaplan, 6/e, p 2761.)* A subpoena does not require that the psychiatrist immediately surrender the psychiatric records. It cannot be enforced until there is an opportunity to appear before a judge in a hearing. This offers an opportunity to present arguments such as belief that the release of the information will be destructive to the patient or the family. By contrast, a court-approved search warrant by law enforcement officers does not provide such an opportunity for challenge.

482. The answer is E. *(Kaplan, 6/e, pp 1720–1722.)* Nancy Cruzan had been in a vegetative state and kept alive by feeding tubes over 4 years. Because her prognosis was hopeless, her parents went to court to have the feeding stopped so that she could die. The case ultimately found its way to the Supreme Court, which ruled that competent persons have a constitutional right to refuse unwanted medical treatment. The court left it to the states to decide how to handle the situation of the incompetent patient, and in many states, that has limited the rights of families to make decisions unless there is an advance directive such as a "living will" and a "durable power of attorney."

483. The answer is C. *(Kaplan, 6/e, p 2764.)* Most U.S. federal courts presently use the American Law Institute (ALI) test, or a minor variation, to determine criminal responsibility. The ALI standard states, "It shall be a defense that the defendant at the time of the proscribed conduct, as a result of mental disease or defect, lacked substantial capacity either to appreciate the wrongfulness of his conduct or to conform his conduct to the requirements of the law." Many jurisdictions have appended a section that states, "The terms mental disease or defect do not include an abnormality manifested only by repeated criminal or otherwise antisocial conduct." This provision is designed to prevent persons with antisocial personalities from offering an insanity defense. Recent decisions in some jurisdictions suggest that the federal judiciary may be moving back toward M'Naghten.

484. The answer is D. *(Kaplan, 6/e, pp 2761–2762.)* Privileged communication must be provided by statute. Where the privilege exists, it is essentially "owned" by the person whose medical information is being sought. Persons may waive the privilege and allow their psychiatrists to testify. Because there are many qualifications to statutory privilege, some feel that the concept is almost meaningless.

485. The answer is D. *(Kaplan, 6/e, pp 2761–2762.)* The Tarasoff decision was a landmark case in determining that psychotherapists have an obligation to warn third parties who are in danger. In this instance, the therapist had an obligation to warn the potential victim of a student who had threatened to kill the girl who had rejected him. He ultimately killed her, and thus began the litigation.

486-487. The answers are 486-B, 487-A. *(Kaplan, 6/e, p 2755.)* Persons have the right to bequeath their estates to any persons or institutions of their choice. However, for their last will and testament to be valid, they must have testamentary capacity. There is no requirement that they be free of the diagnosis of psychiatric disorder, but testamentary capacity does involve several important criteria. Testators must know who their relatives are and who may have claim to their estate. They must have a reasonable estimate of the extent of their assets, know they are signing a will, and understand the meaning of that act. Undue influence may be grounds for invalidating part or all of a will if it can be shown that the influence was sufficient to lead the testator to make decisions he or she might not otherwise have made. Undue influence relates to voluntariness rather than cognitive capacity and is a distinct and important concept in evaluating a will.

488. The answer is B. *(Kaplan, 6/e, p 2749.)* Suicide is the most common reason for malpractice claims to be filed against psychiatrists. This is consistent with the fact that suicide engenders the worst feelings in surviving family members. Appropriate risk management includes careful and documented appraisal of suicidal risk, appropriate assessment and monitoring of the patient, and active involvement with the family.

489. The answer is B. *(Kaplan, 6/e, p 2755.)* Patients are increasingly aware and concerned about who will make decisions for them if they lose the ability to make their own decisions. This might be from a recurrent mental illness such as bipolar disorder, a medical illness, or later-life vegetative states. The durable power of attorney allows the selection of a decision maker in advance who can then act without the necessity of a court proceeding.

490. The answer is A. *(Kaplan, 6/e, p 2757.)* There is no legal obligation to accept any patient for therapy, but once the doctor-patient relationship is established, there are legal and ethical obligations on the doctor to keep informed about the patient's condition and to provide needed care. Abandonment that results in injury may establish grounds for malpractice. The safety and welfare of the patient is paramount. To simply provide medication does not account for the fact that the patient may decompensate and injure himself during the period of time it takes to find a new psychiatrist. The therapist may terminate treatment with an uncooperative or noncompliant patient, but only if assistance is given in finding a new therapist.

491. The answer is E. *(Kaplan, 6/e, pp 2752–2753.)* Informed consent is a matter of both ethics and law. It reflects respect for the patient's autonomy as a person who can reason and make decisions about his or her personal welfare. The courts have upheld these principles, and federal grants are very explicit in their requirements for informed consent. Many drug studies involve the use of placebos. While the patient is informed that placebos are given as part of the research design, it is not required that the physician disclose when the patient is taking active medication versus placebo.

492. The answer is D. *(Kaplan, 6/e, pp 2761–2762.)* Tarasoff-I held that psychotherapists and the police have a duty to warn third parties who are in danger. Tarasoff-II stated that once a therapist has reasonably determined that a patient poses a serious danger of violence to others, he "bears a duty to exercise reasonable care to protect the foreseeable victim of that danger." This is an expansion of the more narrow duty to warn. It also exempted the police from liability. There is no explicit requirement for specific treatment, such as medications or hospitalization, though these might well be employed by the psychiatrist in the management of potentially violent persons.

493. The answer is D. *(Kaplan, 6/e, p 2773.)* In "The Principles of Medical Ethics with Annotations Especially Applicable to Psychiatry," the American Psychiatric Association (APA) unequivocally states that sexual activity with patients is unethical. Such activity is viewed as a misuse and exploitation of the transference relationship, which may activate sexual feelings in both patient and therapist. Psychiatrists have been prosecuted for rape in a few instances, loss of licensure or other licensure action is not uncommon, and malpractice suits with substantial settlements are increasingly common.

While some have advocated that a "waiting period" of a year might be a reasonable way to approach this ethical issue, the APA has pointed out that the transference may persist long after treatment ends.

494. The answer is B. *(Kaplan, 6/e, p 2761.)* Privilege is a right that belongs to the patient, not to the doctor. It is not time-limited and therefore does not end no matter how long it has been since the doctor last saw the patient. The clinician may be ordered by the court to divulge information ordinarily considered privileged, and a patient loses the privilege if suing the doctor or if the patient is claiming emotional harm as a part of a lawsuit against someone. Many jurisdictions consider information relative to child-custody decisions to lie outside privilege.

495–500. The answers are 495-E, 496-A, 497-D, 498-C, 499-C, 500-B. *(Kaplan, 6/e, p 2763.)* The AMA has recommended, and some states have codified, that the insanity defense be abolished. There is considerable question as to whether this can be done constitutionally. Such attempts often direct that the psychiatrist should testify only as to the mens rea elements in criminal trials. This is testimony that addresses the issue of whether the defendant possessed a criminal intent or state of mind at the time of the crime.

In 1843 Daniel M'Naghten was accused of killing the secretary of the Prime Minister of Great Britain. He was acquitted on grounds of insanity, and public outrage led to the development of the M'Naghten test regarding criminal insanity. It is a test primarily related to cognitive functions. It became the test of insanity in many jurisdictions in the United States and is still retained by some states.

The Durham rule, a 1954 decision by the District of Columbia Circuit Court, eliminated the cognitive issues that were associated with the M'Naghten rule, as well as the concept of irresistible impulse that had expanded it in some jurisdictions in order to introduce the concept of volitional control over one's behavior. It gave wide latitude to psychiatric testimony. It was rejected in 1972 because there was simply too much variation in psychiatric opinion as to what constituted the "product of mental disease or mental defect."

The Model Penal Code developed by the American Law Institute (ALI) did not attempt to define mental disease or defect, but it did specify that "the terms 'mental disease' or 'defect' do not include an abnormality manifested only by repeated criminal or otherwise antisocial conduct." This reflected the opinion that sociopaths should not be able to evade criminal responsibility for their acts by claiming that their behavior was on the basis of their psychiatric problem.

Most federal circuit courts and approximately 25 states have adopted at least parts of the rule developed by the ALI. The rule has at least some elements of cognitive (M'Naghten) and volitional (irresistible impulse) determinations. However, it is no longer an issue of "all or nothing." The word "appreciate," for example, acknowledges that a psychotic person may "know" right from wrong, but may lack an ability to truly comprehend the substance and consequences of the behavior. Consider the case of a psychotic who knows that murder is morally and legally wrong, but who kills a neighbor while acting under the influence of paranoid delusions and compelling hallucinations.

Bibliography

American Psychiatric Association: *Diagnostic and Statistical Manual of Mental Disorders,* 4/e (DSM-IV). Washington, DC, American Psychiatric Press, 1994.

American Psychiatric Association: *Practice Guidelines.* Washington, DC, American Psychiatric Press, 1996.

Andreasen, NC, Black, DW: *Introductory Textbook of Psychiatry,* 2/e. Washington, DC, American Psychiatric Press, 1995.

Busse EW, Blazer DG (eds): *American Psychiatric Press Textbook of Geriatric Psychiatry,* 2/e. Washington, DC, American Psychiatric Press, 1996.

Coffey CE, Cummins JL (eds): *American Psychiatric Press Textbook of Geriatric Neuropsychiatry.* Washington, DC, American Psychiatric Press, 1994.

Gabbard GO (ed): *Treatments of Psychiatric Disorders,* 2/e, 2 vols. Washington, DC, American Psychiatric Press, 1995.

Galanter M, Kleber HD (eds): *American Psychiatric Press Textbook of Substance Abuse Treatment.* Washington, DC, American Psychiatric Press, 1994.

Hales RE, Yudofsky SC, Talbott JA (eds): *American Psychiatric Press Textbook of Psychiatry,* 2/e. Washington, DC, American Psychiatric Press, 1994.

Hardman JG, Limbird LE, Molinoff PB, et al (eds): *Goodman and Gilman's The Pharmacological Basis of Therapeutics,* 9/e. New York, McGraw-Hill, 1996.

Isselbacher KJ, Braunwald E, Wilson JD, et al (eds): *Harrison's Principles of Internal Medicine,* 13/e. New York, McGraw-Hill, 1994.

Kaplan HI, Sadock BJ (eds): *Comprehensive Textbook of Psychiatry,* 6/e, 2 vols. Baltimore, Williams & Wilkins, 1995.

Nemiroff RA, Colarusso CA: *New Dimensions in Adult Development.* New York, Basic Books, 1990.

Nersessian E, Kopff Jr RG (eds): *American Psychiatric Press Textbook of Psychoanalysis.* Washington, DC, American Psychiatric Press, 1996.

Rundell JR, Wise MG (eds): *American Psychiatric Press Textbook of Consultation-Liaison Psychiatry.* Washington, DC, American Psychiatric Press, 1996.

Schatzberg AF, Nemiroff CB (eds): *American Psychiatric Press Textbook of Psychopharmacology.* Washington, DC, American Psychiatric Press, 1995.

Schuckit MA: *Drug and Alcohol Abuse: A Clinical Guide to Diagnosis and Treatment* 4/e. New York, Plenum, 1995.

Yudofsky SC, Hales RE (eds): *American Psychiatric Press Textbook of Neuropsychiatry,* 2/e. Washington, DC, American Psychiatric Press, 1992.